BBC goodfood eatwell

SUPERFOOD RECIPES

EDITOR
Cassie Best

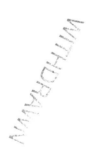

BBC
BOOKS

10 9 8 7 6 5 4 3 2 1

BBC Books, an imprint of Ebury Publishing
20 Vauxhall Bridge Road,
London SW1V 2SA

BBC Books is part of the Penguin Random House
group of companies whose addresses can be
found at:
global.penguinrandomhouse.com

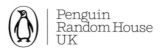

Penguin
Random House
UK

First published by BBC Books in 2017

www.penguin.co.uk

A CIP catalogue record for this book is available
from the British Library

ISBN 9781785941955   641.5637

Printed and bound in China by C&C
Offset Printing Co., Ltd

Typeset in India by Integra Software Services Pvt. Ltd

Project editor: Grace Paul
Cover Design: Interstate Creative Partners Ltd
Production: Alex Goddard
Picture Researchers: Gabby Harrington

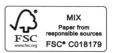

PICTURE AND RECIPE CREDITS

BBC *Good Food* Magazine and BBC Books would like
to thank the following for providing photographs.
While every effort has been made to trace and
acknowledge all photographers, we should like to
apologise should there be any errors or omissions.

Mike English p13, p21, p23, p27, p31, p37, p39, p45,
p67, p87, p89, p95, p113, p113, p135, p143, p159, p165,
p167, p175, p179, p181, p199, p203, p205, p209, p211,
p219, p221, p225, p227, p241, p273, p277, p281, p291,
p301, p303, p305; Peter Cassidy p25, p51, p55, p57,
p61, p69, p131, p187, p257, p269; Helen Cathcart
p47; Will Heap p59, p115, p123, p177, p232, p247,
p253, p309; Jonathan Kennedy p249; Kris Kirkham
p109, p125; Adrian Lawrence p267, p307; Alex Luck
p103; David Munns p35, p53, p91, p127, p173, p201;
Stuart Ovenden p11, p33, p63, p85, p145, p161, p213,
p223, p229, p239, p289, p297, p299; Lis Parsons p251,
p261, p283; Tom Regester p9, p15, p29, p111, p147,
p151, p157, p191, p193, p207, p235, p245, p255; Toby
Scott p49, p65, p149, p153, p163; Simon Smith p71,
p313; Sam Stowell p41, p73, p138, p155, p171, p185,
p237, p259, p279, p285, p295, p311, p317; Rob
Streeter p17, p77, p83, p97, p99, p101, p107, p117, p119,
p169, p183, p189, p195, p216, p275; Philip Webb p93,
p121, p136, p293; Jon Whitaker p263; Clare Winfield
p19, p79, p81, p129, p243, p315

All the recipes in this book were created by the
editorial team at *Good Food* and by regular
contributors to BBC Magazines.

Contents

Introduction

Although it's a familiar term it may come as a surprise that there's no official definition of a 'superfood'. When asked most people would name an exotic fruit or berry but in fact there are plenty of fabulous foods, native to our climate, which nutritionally add a super boost to a healthy, balanced diet.

For us at *BBC Good Food* 'superfoods' are those nutrient-dense foods that supply one or more of the key macronutrients (protein, fats, carbohydrates) whilst also being abundant with antioxidants, minerals, vitamins and phyto-chemicals. These superfoods have the power to improve your health by reducing inflammation, aiding blood flow and boosting immunity. It's important to remember there's no one food that is the answer to long and sustained good health – the greater the variety of the foods you eat the more likely it is that you will be getting all the nutrients your body needs to function at its very best.

Fruit and veg, and especially veg are the foundation of any superfood diet. Eating as wide a selection as possible is key and that is why we encourage you to eat the rainbow. All the wonderful colours represent the different antioxidants and phyto-chemicals that the fruit and veg contain, including anthocyanins, polyphenols, flavonoids and carotenoids. These compounds protect against modern day diseases, but each in a slightly different way. That's why we've devoted three chapters to the rainbow of fruit and vegetables, which can benefit health from better moods to a strengthened immunity. You'll find all of our superfood recipes (not just the three rainbow chapters) loaded with fruit and vegetables, helping you achieve the recommended 5 a day plus.

We've made sure that the following recipes are a balanced combination of protein, fats and carbs, this helps balance hormones and blood sugar, regulating your mood and controlling your appetite. Fat and carbs have had a bad press of late but they are both essential components of a balanced, superfood diet.

Most of the foods we eat supply some fat be they meat, fish, nuts, seeds and grains or dairy and eggs. Our recipes include full fat rather than processed low-fat ingredients, such as yogurt, and extra virgin cold-pressed oils rather than refined ones. That's because all fats are not equal – we should avoid processed, refined fats and oils and limit our intake of saturated varieties. That said there are some saturated fats that are valuable to a superfood diet, more of which later.

For energizing carbs we've focused on the complex variety in the form of whole-grains as well as beans and pulses. Studies suggest eating three or more portions of whole-grains a day can have significant benefits for the heart. It's not difficult to achieve – start your day with porridge for breakfast (page 78) quinoa salad (page 56) for lunch and a pilaf for supper (page 102).

All of our recipes have been chosen for their health-giving ingredients, whether that's memory-boosting turmeric or stamina-enhancing beetroot. So whether you dip in and out of this book or use it as the basis of your eating plan you can be assured of delicious, nourishing, tried and tested recipes, which will work time and time again. Although superfood eating is about health and wellbeing that doesn't mean you have to sacrifice flavour. We've used ingredients like chorizo and bacon, in moderation, because these add flavour and depth to a dish.

So whether you're looking to improve your health, lose a few pounds or just want to feel lighter and brighter our superfood recipes have the power to help you achieve your goal. What's more all of the recipes have been nutritionally analysed per serving, so you can see at a glance the contribution they'll be making to your super new diet.

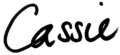

Cassie Best, Editor

Notes & Conversion Tables

NOTES ON THE RECIPES
- Eggs are large in the UK and Australia and extra large in America unless stated.
- Wash fresh produce before preparation.
- Recipes contain nutritional analyses for 'sugar', which means the total sugar content including all natural sugars in the ingredients, unless otherwise stated.

APPROXIMATE WEIGHT CONVERSIONS
- Cup measurements, which are used in Australia and America, have not been listed here as they vary from ingredient to ingredient. Kitchen scales should be used to measure dry/solid ingredients.

Good Food is concerned about sustainable sourcing and animal welfare. Where possible, humanely reared meats, sustainably caught fish (see fishonline.org for further information from the Marine Conservation Society) and free-range chickens and eggs are used when recipes are originally tested.

APPROXIMATE LIQUID CONVERSIONS

Metric	Imperial	AUS	US
50ml	2fl oz	¼ cup	¼ cup
125ml	4fl oz	½ cup	½ cup
175ml	6fl oz	¾ cup	¾ cup
225ml	8fl oz	1 cup	1 cup
300ml	10fl oz/½ pint	½ pint	1¼ cups
450ml	16fl oz	2 cups	2 cups/1 pint
600ml	20fl oz/1 pint	1 pint	2½ cups
1 litre	35fl oz/1¾ pints	1¾ pints	1 quart

OVEN TEMPERATURES

GAS°C	°C FAN	°F	OVEN TEMP.
¼ 110	90	225	Very cool
½ 120	100	250	Very cool
1 140	120	275	Cool or slow
2 150	130	300	Cool or slow
3 160	140	325	Warm
4 180	160	350	Moderate
5 190	170	375	Moderately hot
6 200	180	400	Fairly hot
7 220	200	425	Hot
8 230	210	450	Very hot
9 240	220	475	Very hot

SPOON MEASURES
Spoon measurements are level unless otherwise specified.
- 1 teaspoon (tsp) = 5ml
- 1 tablespoon (tbsp) = 15ml
- 1 Australian tablespoon = 20ml (cooks in Australia should measure 3 teaspoons where 1 tablespoon is specified in a recipe)

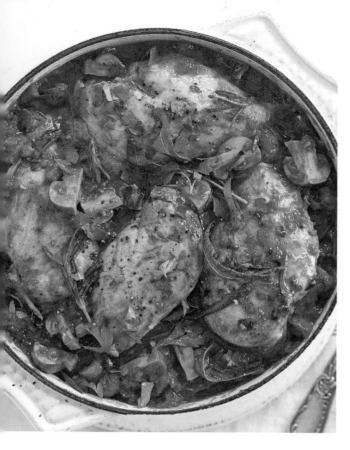
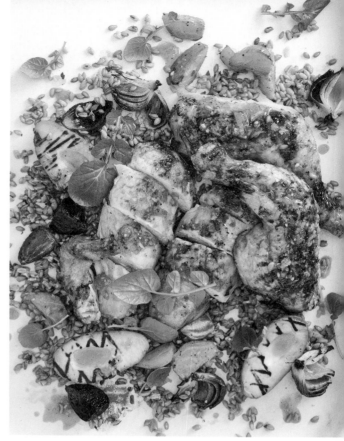
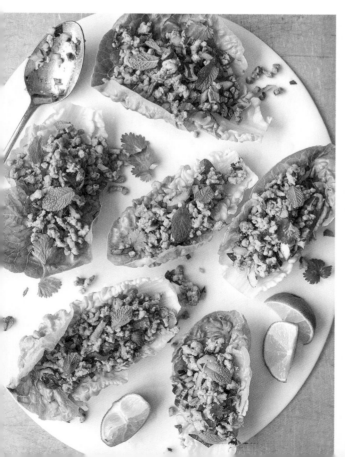
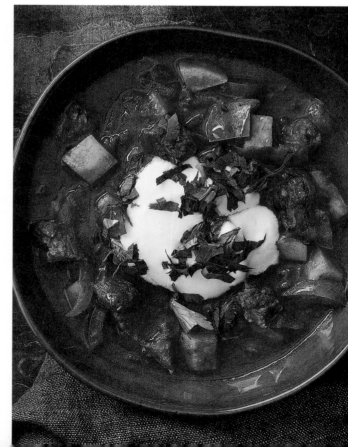

Chapter 1:

POWERFUL PROTEIN

....

Essential for every cell in the body, not to mention the function of hormones, nerves and enzymes; protein forms the building blocks for strong muscles, beautiful skin and hair. Protein is an essential part of a balanced diet because we all have an ongoing need for it – the average woman needing about 50-60g per day.

By including protein, in the form of fish, poultry, lean red meat, dairy and eggs at each meal you'll be providing the essential building blocks known as amino acids. A protein source is said to be a *complete* protein when it supplies all the essential amino acids in the required proportions. Lean red meat can play an important part in a superfood diet because as well as being a complete protein it's loaded with iron, a mineral that many women are low in.

For those with weight loss as a goal, protein makes a smart choice because your body uses more calories digesting it than it does for fats and carbs.

What's more studies have shown that by enjoying a protein-rich breakfast you'll feel fuller for longer and eat fewer calories later in the day. So forget that carb-rich bowl of cereal and opt for eggs like our Superfood scrambled eggs (page 14). That said, you don't have to eat a substantial meal – a bowl of bone broth is nourishing, yet filling. Rich in amino acids and collagen, a bowl of broth will support beautiful nails, skin and hair. Try our delicious version on page 36.

Whether you're a vegetarian or a committed meat-eater, plant-based sources of protein are a must – include soya like tofu, pulses, beans, quinoa, nuts and seeds. We've used quinoa flour in our Protein pancakes (page 8) – it's richer in protein than wheat and supplies energizing B vitamins as well as the muscle-relaxing mineral, magnesium.

Protein pancakes with blueberries & raspberries

Start the day with a protein-packed breakfast, loaded with extra goodness from blueberries, seeds and nuts.

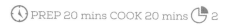 PREP 20 mins COOK 20 mins 2

FOR THE BATTER
- 2 tbsp ground flaxseeds
- 20g ground almonds
- 300ml soya milk
- 200g quinoa flour
- 1 medium banana, mashed
- 2 tbsp maple syrup
- coconut oil, for frying

FOR THE BLUEBERRY CHIA JAM (MAKES 200ML)
- 200g blueberries, mashed
- 2 tbsp chia seeds
- 1–2 tbsp maple syrup, to taste
- 2 tsp lemon juice

FOR THE STACK
- 100g coconut yogurt or Greek yogurt
- 1 tbsp pistachio nuts or pumpkin seeds, chopped, toasted if you like
- 2 tsp hulled hemp seeds
- mixed berries

1 In a small bowl stir the flaxseeds with 6 tbsp water and set aside to soak while you make the jam.

2 Mash the blueberries with a fork in a pan then set over a low-medium heat until syrupy and bubbling. Remove from the heat and stir in the chia seeds, maple syrup and lemon juice. Leave to cool slightly then transfer to a small serving jar.

3 Put the ground almonds, milk, flour, banana, maple syrup and a pinch of salt in a blender. Stir the flax to make sure it has become thick and gloopy, like an egg, then tip into the mix and blitz until smooth and thick. Heat 1 tsp of coconut oil in a large frying pan over a medium heat and add tablespoon dollops of batter into the pan. Cook for a couple of mins on one side until the edges are browning, and bubbles have formed on top. Once the pale, white batter has turned a sandy colour, flip over with a spatula and cook for another few mins till dark golden brown. Set aside and keep warm while you repeat the process with the remaining batter, adding another tsp of coconut oil with each batch. You should make about 16 pancakes.

4 Pile the pancakes high between two plates, alternating the layers with spoonfuls of jam and yogurt. Dollop any remaining yogurt and another spoonful of jam on top then scatter over the nuts, seeds and berries to serve. Leftover jam will keep in the fridge for up to 1 week.

Nutrition: *per serving*
kcal 798 fat 32g saturates 8g carbs 91g sugars 39g fibre 15g protein 29g salt 0.3g

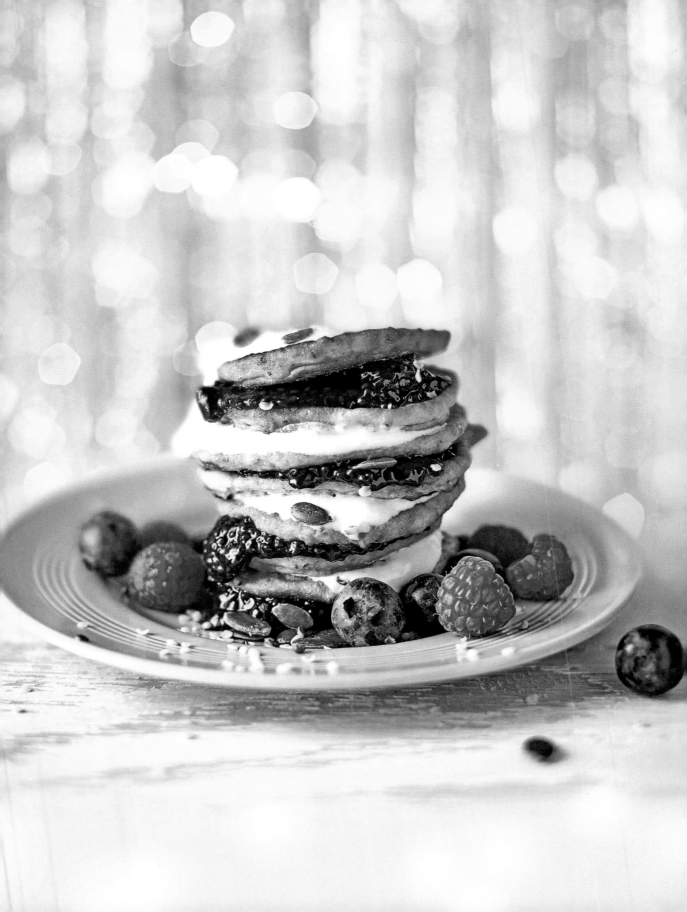

Chicken & avocado salad with blueberry balsamic dressing

Women can enjoy over half their daily recommended intake of protein with this easy chicken salad.

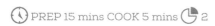 PREP 15 mins COOK 5 mins 2

- 1 garlic clove
- 85g blueberries
- 1 tbsp extra virgin rapeseed oil
- 2 tsp balsamic vinegar
- 125g fresh or frozen baby broad beans
- 1 large cooked beetroot, finely chopped
- 1 avocado, stoned, peeled and sliced
- 85g bag mixed baby leaf salad
- 175g cooked chicken

1 Finely chop the garlic. Mash half the blueberries with the oil, vinegar and some black pepper in a large salad bowl.
2 Boil the broad beans for 5 mins until just tender. Drain, leaving them unskinned.
3 Stir the garlic into the dressing, then pile in the warm beans and remaining blueberries with the beetroot, avocado, salad and chicken. Toss to mix, but don't go overboard or the juice from the beetroot will turn everything pink. Pile onto plates or into shallow bowls to serve.

Nutrition: *per serving*
kcal 402 fat 19g saturates 3g carbs 18g sugars 10g fibre 10g protein 34g salt 0.3g

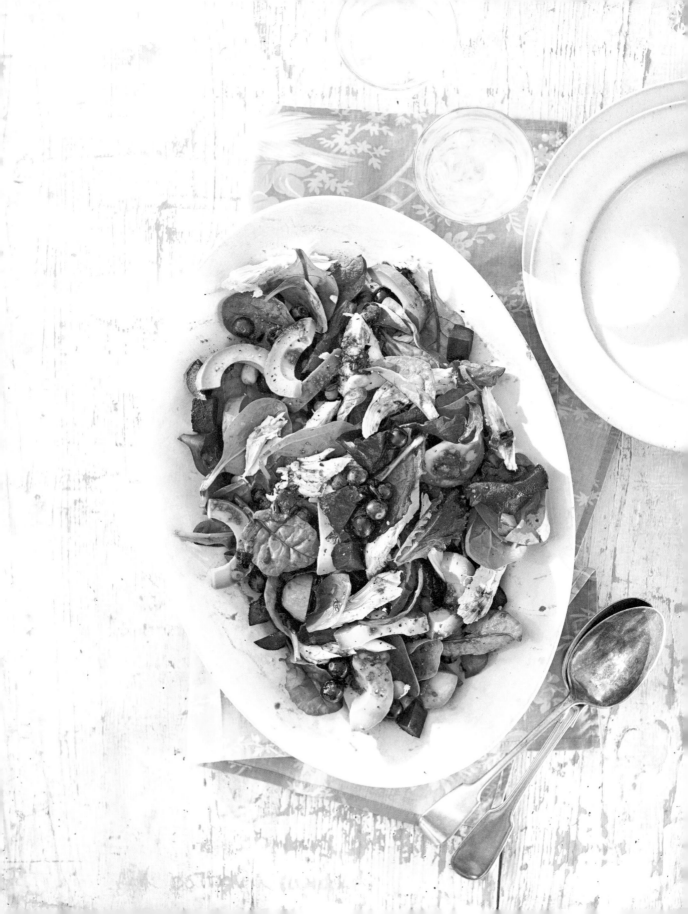

Blackened salmon fajitas

This super-speedy dinner will see you on your way to hitting your protein target for the day. Add some sliced, stir-fried peppers to the wraps to increase your fruit and veg intake, if you like.

PREP 5 mins COOK 8 mins 4

- 4 salmon fillets
- sunflower oil, or any oil suitable for frying
- 2 tbsp fajita spice mix
- 8 tortilla wraps
- 2 avocados
- 2 limes
- 4 tbsp salsa

1 Coat the salmon in 1 tbsp oil and the fajita spice mix. Add 1 tbsp oil to a frying pan and fry 3-4 mins each side, until cooked through and charred in places.
2 Warm the tortillas to packet instructions. Mash the avocados with a fork, season and squeeze over the juice of 1 lime. Serve the salmon in large flakes with the tortillas, avocado, salsa and the other lime, cut into wedges.

Nutrition: *per serving*
kcal 759 fat 45g saturates 10g carbs 46g sugars 8g fibre 7g protein 39g salt 2g

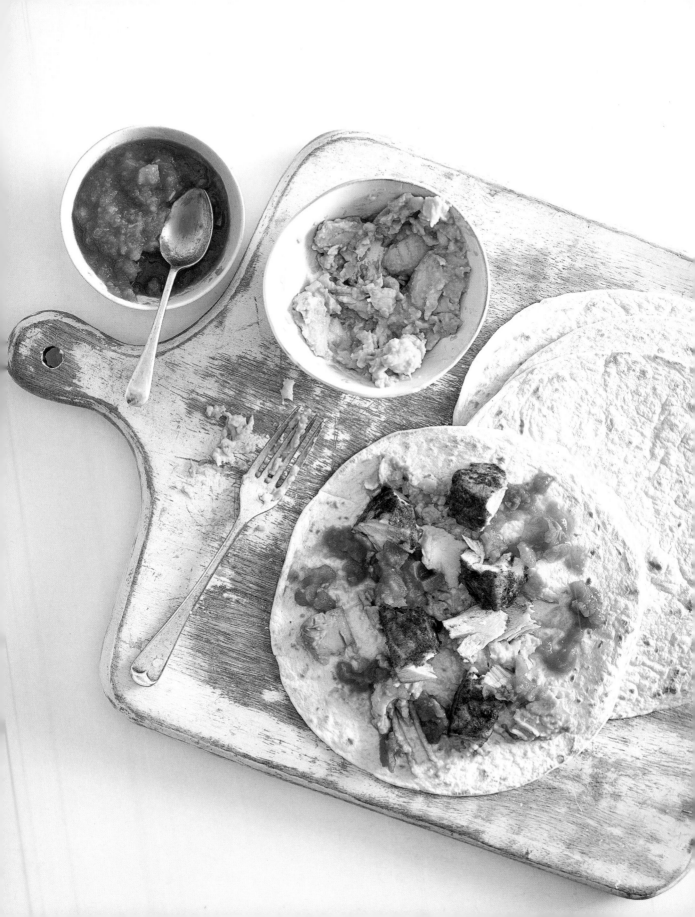

Superfood scrambled eggs

Give up your sugary breakfast cereal in favour of this nutrient-dense breakfast.

PREP 3 mins COOK 7 mins 2

- 2 tbsp pumpkin seeds
- 2 tsp extra virgin rapeseed oil
- 100g spinach, roughly chopped
- 1 tomato, chopped
- 1 garlic clove, crushed
- ½ tsp turmeric
- ½ tsp curry powder
- 4 eggs, beaten
- 150g smoked salmon
- toast, to serve (optional)

1 Tip the pumpkin seeds into a saucepan and toast over a high heat until they start to pop, then transfer to a plate.
2 Add the oil to the pan along with the spinach, tomato and garlic. Cook for 1–2 mins until the spinach has wilted, then add the turmeric, curry powder and eggs. Scramble the eggs over a medium heat – take the pan off the heat before they look too dry. Serve with the pumpkin seeds and the salmon, on toast, if you like.

Nutrition: *per serving*
kcal 409 fat 26g saturates 5g carbs 5g sugars 2g fibre 2g protein 38g salt 2g

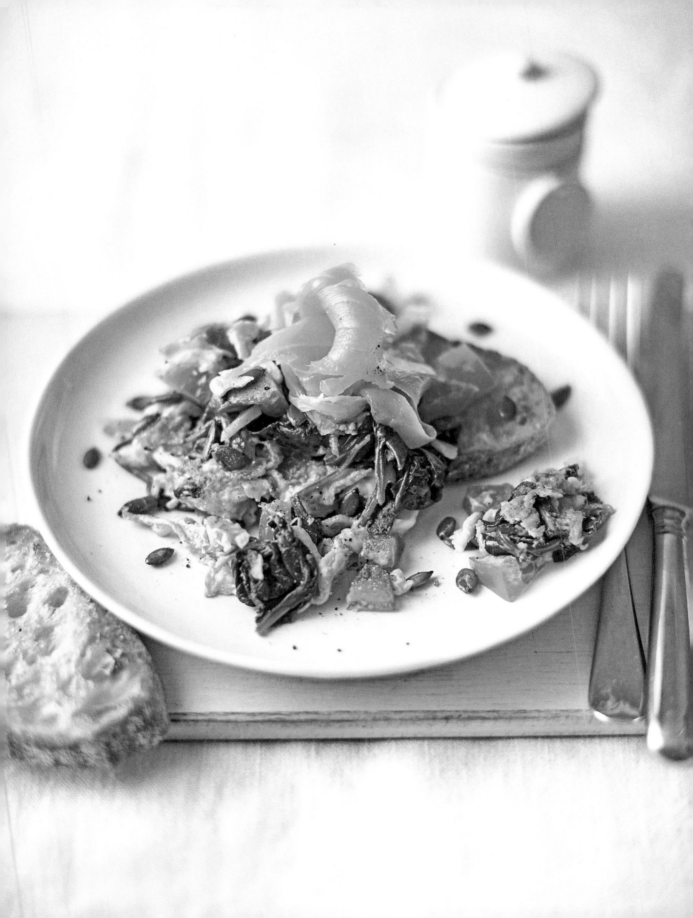

Fresh & light chowder

This dish makes an easy, light supper. Perfect for those nights when you want something hearty but low in calories.

🕐 PREP 10 mins COOK 40 mins 🥧 4

- 100g smoked haddock fillets and 100g unsmoked, skin on
- 500ml whole milk
- 500ml vegetable stock
- 2 thyme sprigs
- 1 tsp vegetable oil
- 1 onion, finely chopped
- 1 garlic clove, finely chopped
- 1 leek, sliced
- 1 large sweet potato, diced
- 200g can sweetcorn in water, drained
- 50g red lentils
- small handful celery leaves or parsley, chopped
- crusty brown bread, to serve

1 Place the fish in a deep frying pan, then add the milk, stock and thyme. Bring to the boil and take off the heat; leave until cool enough to handle. Take out the fish (reserving the liquid), peel off the skin and flake the fish onto a plate, to use later.

2 Meanwhile, heat the oil in a large saucepan. Gently fry the onion, garlic and leek for 8–10 mins until soft and translucent. Add the sweet potato, sweetcorn and lentils, then pour over the liquid you cooked the fish in. Bring to the boil and simmer for 30 mins. Check the seasoning and semi-blitz with a hand blender, leave it quite rough. Add the flaked fish and chopped parsley. Serve piping hot with some crusty bread.

Nutrition: *per serving*
kcal 303 fat 6g saturates 3g carbs 38g sugars 15g fibre 6g protein 20g salt 1.3g

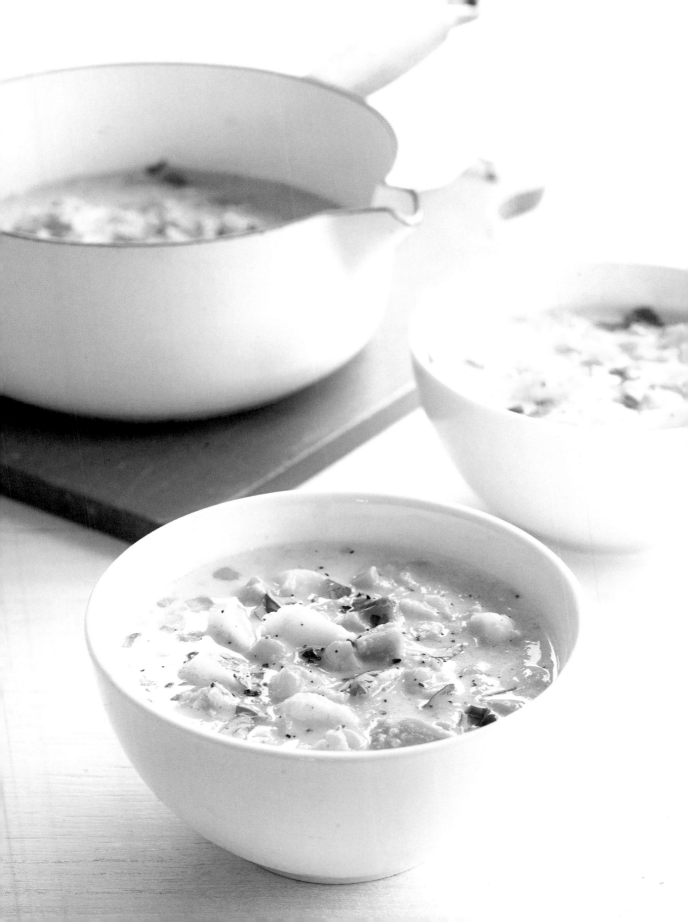

Ham, spinach & mushroom frittata

Breakfast, lunch or dinner, this is a nutritious dish for any time of day. Leftovers also travel well in a lunchbox and are delicious cold.

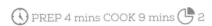 PREP 4 mins COOK 9 mins 2

- 1 tsp oil
- 80g chestnut mushrooms, sliced
- 50g ham, diced
- 80g bag spinach
- 4 medium eggs, beaten
- 1 tbsp grated cheddar

1 Heat the grill to its highest setting. Heat the oil in an ovenproof frying pan over a medium-high heat. Tip in the mushrooms and fry for 2 mins until mostly softened. Stir in the ham and spinach, and cook for 1 min more until the spinach has wilted. Season well with black pepper and a pinch of salt.

2 Reduce the heat and pour over the eggs. Cook undisturbed for 3 mins until the eggs are mostly set. Sprinkle over the cheese and put under the grill for 2 mins. Serve hot or cold.

Nutrition: *per serving*
kcal 226 fat 15g saturates 5g carbs 0g sugars 0g fibre 1g protein 22g salt 1.1g

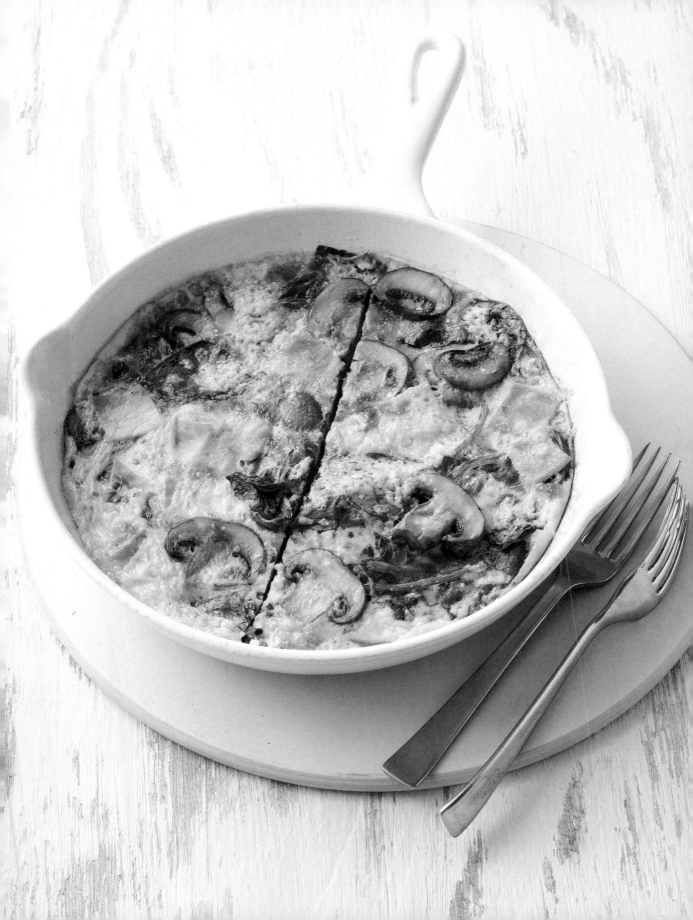

Sticky citrus chicken with griddled avocado & beet salad

· ·

This dish is makes a nice change from your regular Sunday lunch, and with oranges, beetroot and watercress in the mix, also covers off most of the rainbow.

PREP 15 mins COOK 1 hr 4

- 1 chicken (about 1.3kg) spatchcocked (ask the butcher to do this for you, or visit www.bbcgoodfood.com to watch a video)
- 2 red onions, each cut into 8 wedges
- 6 beetroots (a mixture of colours is nice), peeled and each cut into 8 wedges
- 1 tbsp olive oil or rapeseed oil
- 250g spelt
- 2 large, firm avocados
- 100g bag watercress
- natural yogurt, to serve (optional)

FOR THE MARINADE
- 1 small preserved lemon (skin only, discard the middle)
- 4 garlic cloves, crushed
- 2 tsp sweet paprika, plus a pinch
- zest and juice 2 large lemons
- zest and juice 2 large oranges
- 6 tbsp clear honey
- 3 tbsp olive oil or rapeseed oil

1 Make a few slashes in each leg joint of the chicken. Put the chicken in a large sealable plastic bag, or a dish. Now, make the marinade. Rinse the preserved lemon, finely chop the peel until it resembles a paste. Tip into a bowl and add the remaining marinade ingredients and a pinch of salt. Mix, then pour roughly half the marinade over the chicken and rub it into all the nooks. For the best flavour, leave the chicken to marinate overnight, covered, in the fridge (store the remaining marinade in the fridge too), if you're short on time, 2 hrs marinating will do.

2 Heat oven to 200C/180C fan/gas 6. Tip the onions and beetroot into a large roasting tin, drizzle with oil and season well. Place the chicken on top, skin-side up, and pour over any juices from the bag or dish. Season the chicken well and roast for 45 mins.

3 Meanwhile, bring a pan of water to the boil and add the spelt. Cook for 20 mins or until tender, drain and set aside. Halve each avocado, remove the stones and peel. Chop each piece in half again, if you like. Char the avocado pieces on a hot griddle pan for a few mins – this will give it a smoky flavour.

4 Remove the remaining marinade from the fridge and very gently toss the avocado pieces in it, then set them aside. Pour the remaining marinade into a small pan and bring to a rapid boil, then continue cooking for 2–3 mins until you have a sticky glaze.

5 Lift the chicken onto a plate or board and stir the spelt into the vegetables. Place the chicken back on top, dot the avocado pieces around the tin and brush the thickened glaze over the chicken. Return to the oven for a further 5–10 mins. To check the chicken is cooked, pierce the thickest part with a skewer. The juices should run clear, not pink. If you need to, return the chicken to the oven for a further 5–10 mins, then check again.

6 Lift the chicken onto a plate, cover loosely with foil and return the roasting tin with the vegetables to the oven for a further 10 mins until the avocado starts to soften. To serve, nestle the chicken back into the tin of veg, scatter over a few small watercress leaves and serve the rest on the side with the yogurt.

· ·

Nutrition: *per serving*
kcal 1020 fat 51g saturates 10g carbs 77g sugars 40g fibre 16g protein 55g salt 0.5g

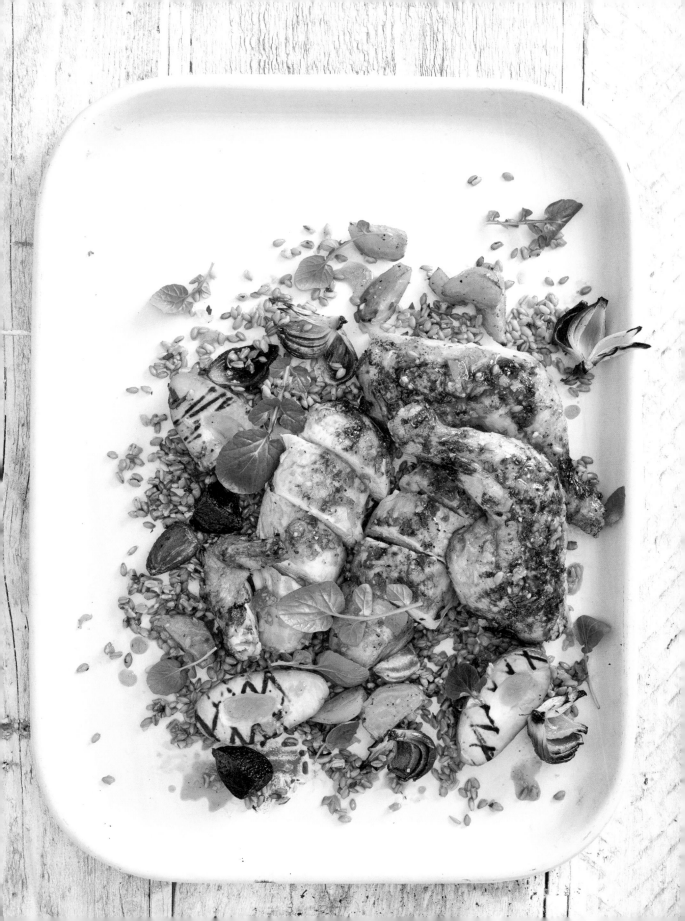

Lighter chicken cacciatore

A lighter version of a classic Italian chicken dish, this translates as Hunter's chicken. Serve it with mashed sweet potatoes and steamed greens, if you like.

PREP 15 mins COOK 50 mins 4

- 1 tbsp olive oil
- 3 slices prosciutto, fat removed, chopped
- 1 medium onion, chopped
- 2 garlic cloves, finely chopped
- 2 sage sprigs
- 2 rosemary sprigs
- 4 skinless chicken breasts
- 150ml dry white wine
- 400g can plum tomatoes
- 1 tbsp tomato purée
- 225g chestnut mushrooms, quartered or halved if large
- small handful chopped flat-leaf parsley, to serve

1 Heat the oil in a large non-stick frying pan. Tip in the prosciutto and fry for about 2 mins until crisp. Remove with a slotted spoon, letting any fat drain back into the pan, and set aside. Put the onion, garlic and herbs in the pan and fry for 3–4 mins.

2 Spread the onion out in the pan, then lay the chicken breasts on top. Season with pepper and fry for 5 mins over a medium heat, turning the chicken once, until starting to brown on both sides and the onion is caramelising on the bottom of the pan. Remove the chicken and set aside on a plate. Raise the heat, give it a quick stir and, when sizzling, pour in the wine and let it bubble for 2 mins to reduce slightly.

3 Lower the heat to medium, return the prosciutto to the pan, then stir in the tomatoes (breaking them up with your spoon), tomato purée and mushrooms. Spoon 4 tbsp of water into the empty tomato can, swirl it around, then pour it into the pan. Cover and simmer for 15–20 mins or until the sauce has thickened and reduced slightly, then return the chicken to the pan and cook, uncovered, for about 15 mins or until the chicken is cooked through. Season and scatter over the parsley to serve.

Nutrition: *per serving*
kcal 262 fat 6.2g saturates 1.3g carbs 6.9g sugars 5.2g fibre 2.7g protein 38.7g salt 1g

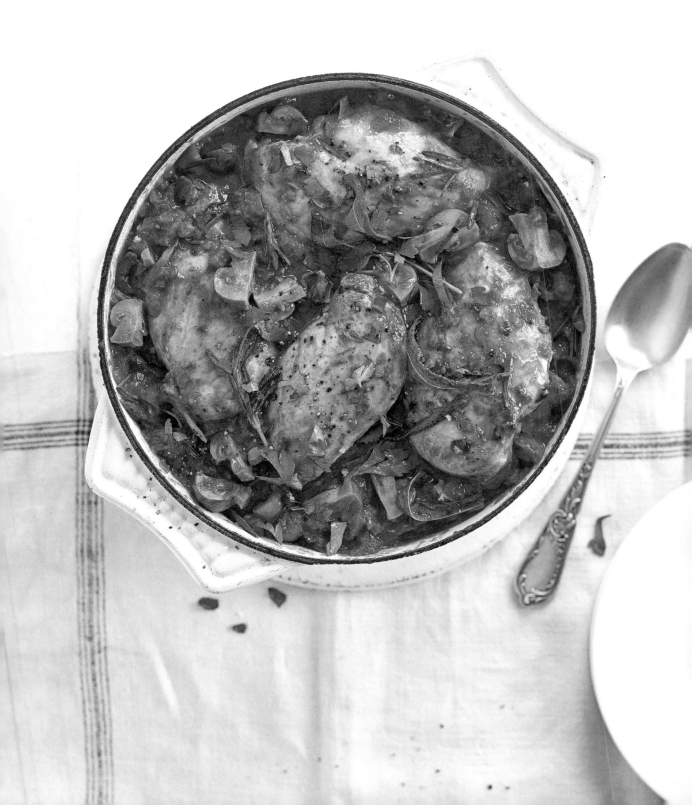

Mexican chicken tortilla soup

This soup is made from a whole chicken, meaning all the goodness, collagen and amino acids (great for healthy skin, hair and nails) from the carcass cooks into the stock.

PREP 40 mins COOK 1 hr 20 mins 8

- 1.2kg whole chicken
- 5 fat red chillies, 4 left whole but pierced a few times with a sharp knife, 1 sliced, to serve
- 2 dried ancho chillies
- 1 garlic bulb, cut in half through the centre horizontally
- bunch coriander, stalks and leaves separated
- 1 cinnamon stick
- 3 tbsp vegetable oil
- 2 large onions, chopped
- 1 tbsp ground cumin
- 1 tbsp ground coriander
- 1 tbsp smoked paprika
- 2 x 400g cans tomatoes
- 1 tsp sugar
- 320g can sweetcorn, drained
- 400g can black beans, drained
- zest and juice 2 limes
- 4 corn tortilla, quartered and cut into strips
- 2 avocados
- 200g feta or queso fresco, crumbled, to serve

1 Put the chicken in a large pan with the whole and dried chillies, garlic, coriander stalks and cinnamon, cover with cold water, then set over a medium heat. When the liquid comes to the boil, reduce to a gentle simmer and cover with a lid. Cook for 30 mins, then turn off the heat and leave the chicken in the stock to cool for 20 mins.

2 Remove the chicken, strain the liquid into a large jug (you should have about 800ml) and discard the aromatics. Return the liquid to the pan and simmer until it has reduced to about 600ml, then pour back into the jug. Heat 1 tbsp oil in the pan, add the onion and cook for 8–10 mins until soft and translucent, then stir in the spices, tomatoes and sugar. Add the chicken stock to the pan, season well and simmer with the lid ajar for 30 mins.

3 While the soup cooks, remove the skin from the chicken and finely shred the meat. Add to the soup along with the sweetcorn, beans, lime zest and juice to taste (save a little to toss through the avocado), and cook for 5 mins more.

4 Heat the remaining oil in a frying pan and add the tortilla pieces. Fry until golden and crispy, then drain on kitchen paper. Halve and peel the avocado, cut into small chunks and toss through the remaining lime juice. Serve the soup in bowls topped with the crispy tortillas, coriander leaves, sliced chilli, avocado and feta.

Nutrition: *per serving*
kcal 483 fat 24g saturates 7g carbs 26g sugars 11g fibre 10g protein 35g salt 1.4g

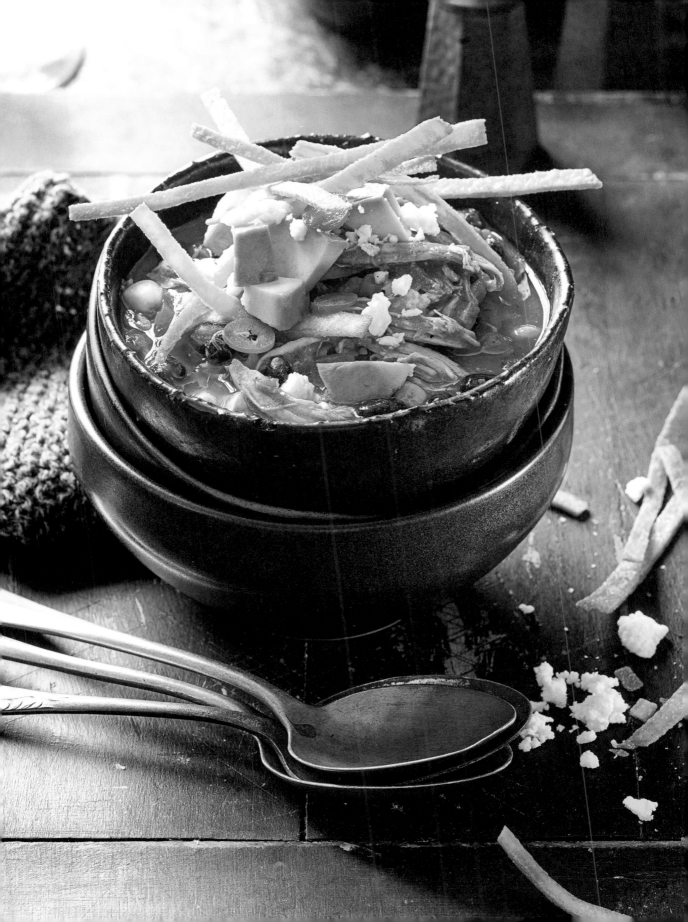

Okonomiyaki

You can add any veg you like to this Japanese pancake, and it's just as good with chicken instead of prawns.

PREP 10 mins COOK 15 mins 1

- 2 slices streaky bacon
- 1 egg
- 50g plain flour
- 50g sweetheart cabbage, finely shredded
- 2 spring onions, sliced diagonally
- 50g small cooked prawns
- 1 tbsp oil
- 1 tsp brown sauce
- 1 tsp mayonnaise

1 Heat a small (about 20cm) non-stick frying pan, add the bacon and cook over a medium-high heat for a few mins until cooked through. Remove the bacon from the pan with a slotted spoon and set aside. Once cool, cut into pieces.

2 Whisk the egg, flour and 4 tbsp water to make a batter, season and stir in the cabbage, half the spring onions, the prawns and the cooked bacon. Pour the oil into the pan, add the mixture and press down, then cook for 5 mins on a medium heat. Flip with a spatula, then cook for another 5 mins until golden and cooked through. Slide onto a plate and drizzle over the brown sauce and mayonnaise. Finally, scatter with the remaining spring onions.

Nutrition: *per serving*
kcal 613 fat 34g saturates 7g carbs 42g sugars 4g fibre 4g protein 33g salt 2.9g

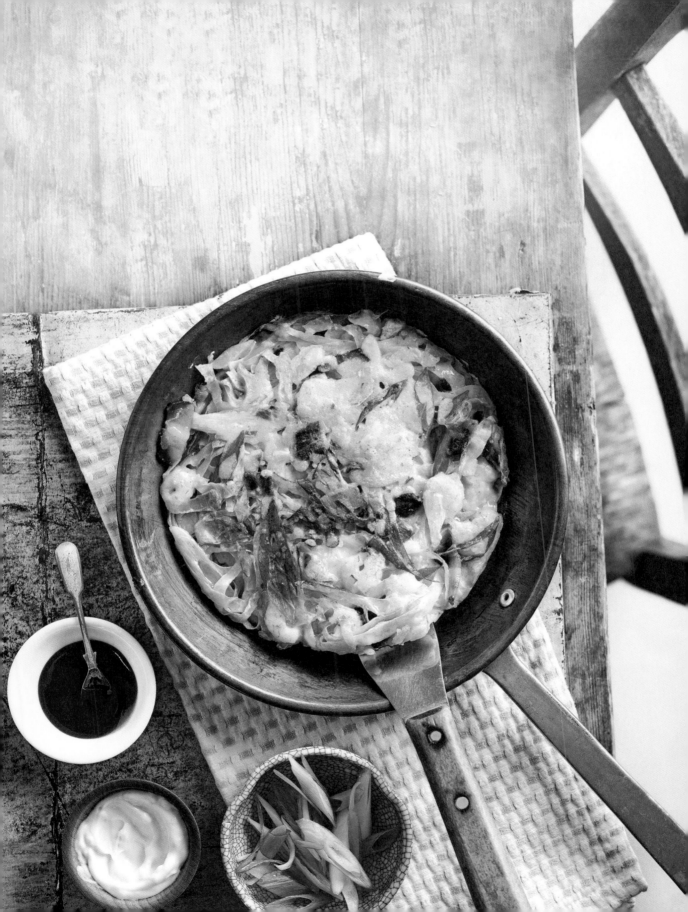

Gado gado salad

This Indonesian salad is packed with interesting flavours and textures. If you want to take this to work in a lunchbox, toss through the dressing just before eating.

PREP 25 mins COOK 15 mins 4–6

- 1 tbsp vegetable oil
- 200g firm tofu, chopped into small chunks
- 250g cooked potatoes (leftover roast potatoes work well), chopped into chunks
- 3 eggs
- 100g green beans, halved lengthways
- 250g Chinese cabbage, finely shredded
- ½ cucumber (or 1 baby cucumber), thinly sliced
- 100g beansprouts
- 1 carrot, shredded
- handful coriander, leaves picked and roughly chopped
- handful prawn crackers
- 4 tbsp crispy onions

FOR THE PEANUT DRESSING
- 50g peanut butter
- 3 tbsp kecap manis (or 2½ tbsp soy sauce and ½ tbsp honey)
- 2 tsp shrimp paste or dried crayfish
- 1 tbsp fish sauce
- 1 tbsp soft dark brown sugar
- 1 garlic clove, crushed
- 2 fat red chillies, finely chopped
- 150ml coconut milk
- juice 1 lime

1 Heat the oil in a large frying pan or wok and boil a small saucepan of water. Fry the tofu for a few mins each side until brown and crispy, then transfer to a plate. Add the potatoes to the frying pan and cook for a few mins until they are warmed through and starting to crisp, then tip onto the same plate and set aside to cool.

2 Add the eggs to the boiling water and cook for 7 mins, then plunge them straight into cold water. Fill the saucepan with fresh water, bring to the boil and add the beans. Cook for 2–3 mins until just tender. Drain and run under cold water until cool.

3 To make the peanut dressing, put the peanut butter and kecap manis in a bowl and mash together with a fork until smooth and combined. Whisk in the remaining ingredients.

4 Put the tofu, potatoes, beans, cabbage, cucumber, beansprouts, carrot and coriander in a large bowl or arrange on a platter. Drizzle over half the dressing, reserving the rest for people to help themselves. Break the prawn crackers in your hands and scatter over. Peel and quarter the eggs, and serve on top with the crispy onions. Toss together just before serving.

Nutrition: *per serving (6)*
kcal 398 fat 22g saturates 6g carbs 30g sugars 13g fibre 4g protein 18g salt 1.5g

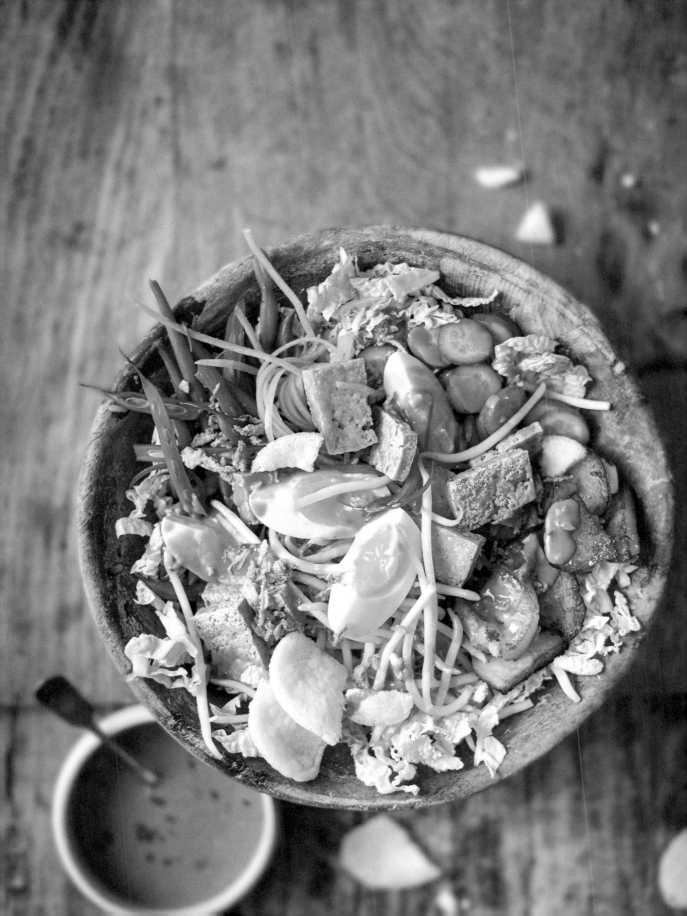

Lemon & fennel pork meatballs

Served from the pot with a loaf of crusty bread for mopping up the sauce, this makes a great comfort food dish for a chilly evening.

PREP 15 mins COOK 40 mins | 4

- 2 tbsp olive oil
- 1 medium onion, finely chopped
- 2 garlic cloves, finely sliced
- 2 x 400g cans plum tomatoes
- 1 lemon, zested and cut into wedges
- 500g pork mince
- 2 tsp fennel seeds
- 250g kale
- 25g pine nuts, toasted
- crusty bread or mashed potato, to serve (optional)

1 In a medium pan, heat 1 tbsp of the oil over a medium heat. Add the onion and garlic to the pan and cook for 5 mins. Tip in the tomatoes with a splash of water, increase the heat and allow to bubble for 15 mins. Meanwhile, in a large bowl, combine the lemon zest, mince, fennel seeds and a good pinch of seasoning. Mix well, then shape into walnut-sized balls.

2 Heat the remaining oil in a lidded frying pan over a medium heat. Add the meatballs and brown for 5 mins, then pour the tomato sauce into the pan. Simmer for 10 mins, then add the kale, cover with a lid and cook for 5 mins more until wilted. Season to taste, and scatter over the pine nuts. Serve with the lemon wedges, for squeezing over, and crusty bread or mash, if you like.

Nutrition: *per serving*
kcal 401 fat 23g saturates 6g carbs 16g sugars 10g fibre 3g protein 31g salt 0.3g

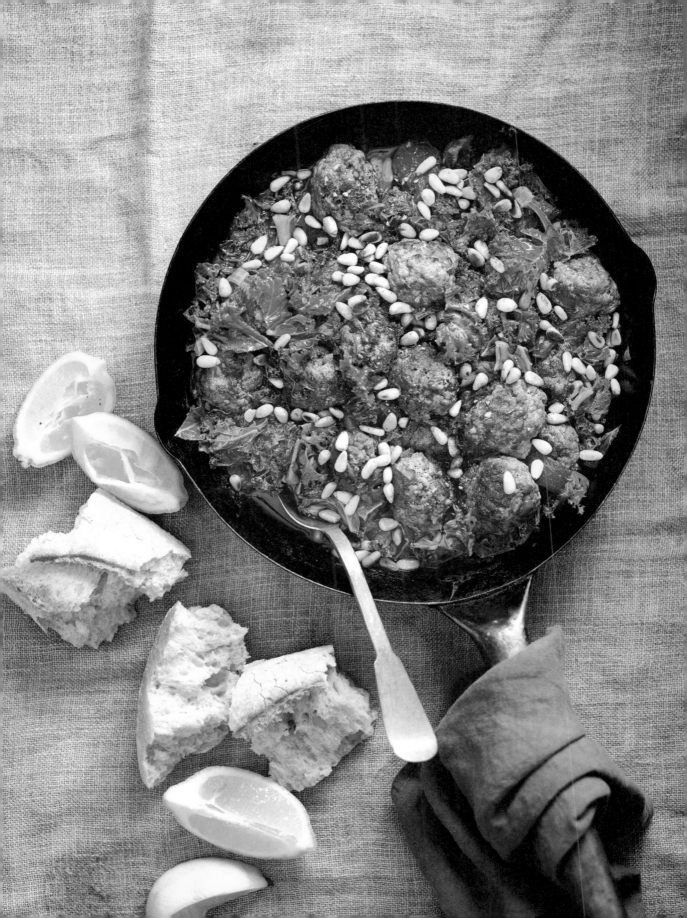

Thai green pork lettuce cups

This dish makes a wonderful lunch or light dinner, or can be served as a canape.

PREP 10 mins COOK 15 mins 4

- 1 tbsp sesame oil
- 500g pork mince
- 1 tbsp green curry paste
- 1 red onion, finely chopped
- juice 1 lime
- 1 tbsp fish sauce
- ½ small pack mint, leaves only, roughly chopped
- ½ small pack coriander, leaves only, roughly chopped
- 4 Little Gem lettuces, leaves separated

1 Heat the oil in a frying pan and cook the pork for 8–10 mins or until cooked through. Stir in the green curry paste and 2 tbsp water, then cook for 1–2 mins.
2 Remove from the heat and stir in the red onion, lime juice, fish sauce and herbs. Spoon the pork into the lettuce leaves and serve with rice, if you like.

Nutrition: *per serving*
kcal 298 fat 17g saturates 5g carbs 7g sugars 6g fibre 3g protein 27g salt 1.1g

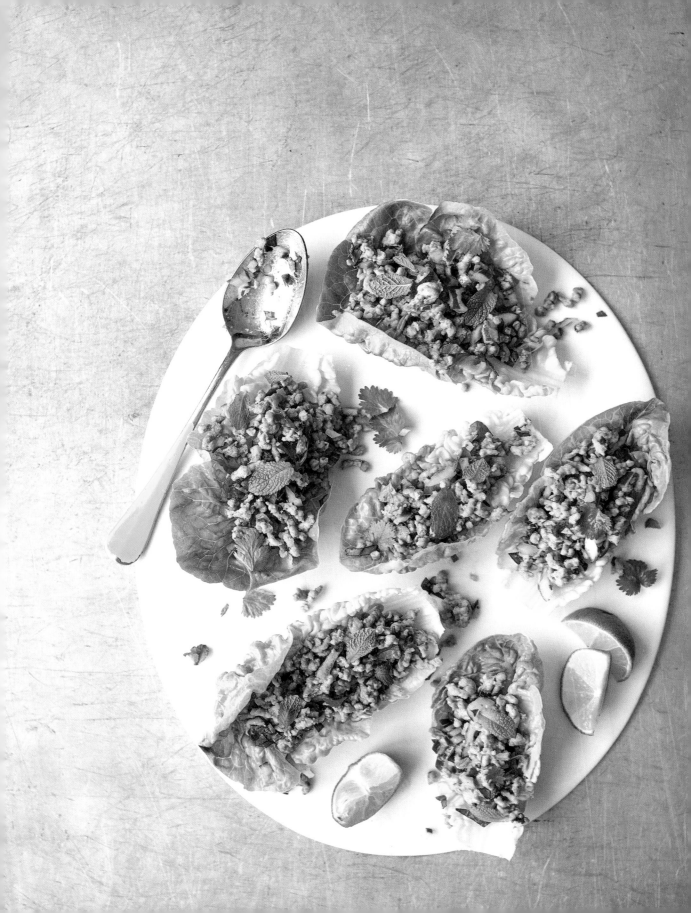

Zingy teriyaki beef skewers

Packed with protein, and rich in iron, this dish is perfect for anyone struggling to get enough iron in their diet.

PREP 20 mins COOK 35 mins plus marinating 2

- 1 tbsp tamari or soy sauce
- 3 tbsp freshly squeezed orange juice
- 15g chunk ginger, peeled and very finely grated
- 2 garlic cloves, crushed
- 1 tsp honey
- ¼ tsp chilli flakes
- 300g beef sirloin steak, trimmed of hard fat and cut into long, thin strips

FOR THE SALAD
- 100g long-grain brown rice
- ⅓ cucumber, cut into small cubes
- 2 medium carrots, peeled and sliced into ribbons with a peeler
- 4 spring onions, trimmed and diagonally sliced
- 100g radishes, trimmed and sliced
- 20g coriander leaves, roughly chopped, plus extra to garnish
- 10g mint leaves, plus extra to garnish
- 1 tbsp extra virgin rapeseed oil
- zest and juice 1 lime
- 25g unsalted cashew nuts, toasted and roughly chopped

1 Put the tamari, orange juice, ginger, garlic, honey and chilli flakes in a small saucepan with 100ml cold water and bring to the boil. Cook for 3–5 mins, boiling hard until well reduced, glossy and slightly syrupy. Remove from the heat, pour into a shallow dish and leave to cool. Thread the beef onto 4 soaked wooden or metal skewers. Place in the marinade, turn and brush until well coated. Cover with cling film and marinate for 30 mins.

2 While the beef is marinating, prepare the salad. Half-fill a medium pan with water and bring to the boil. Cook the rice for about 20 mins or following pack instructions until tender. Rinse in a sieve under running water until cold, then drain well. Tip into a large bowl.

3 Add the cucumber, carrots, spring onions, radishes, coriander, mint, oil, lime zest and juice, and toss together well. Season with a little black pepper. Divide between two plates and top with a sprinkling of nuts and extra herbs to garnish.

4 Heat the grill to high. (You could also cook the skewers on a non-stick griddle pan.) Put the skewers on a rack above a foil-lined baking tray, reserving any excess marinade. Grill the skewers close to the heat for 3–5 mins each side or until done to your liking. Brush with more marinade when they are turned. They should look sticky and glossy when cooked. Serve hot or cold with the rice salad.

Nutrition: *per serving*
kcal 563 fat 22g saturates 6g carbs 46g sugars 16g fibre 9g protein 39g salt 1.4g

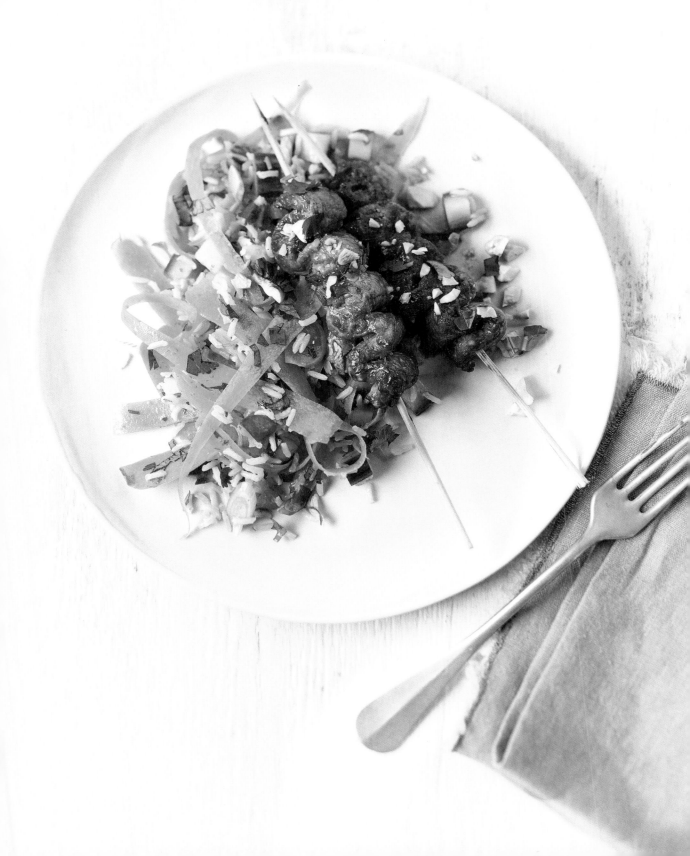

Ramen with bone broth & pork shoulder

This meaty broth takes a few hours to cook, but the result is a rich, hearty soup which will satisfy your taste buds and provide you with plenty of essential nutrients.

🕐 PREP 25 mins COOK 4 hrs 10 mins 🥧 4

- 4 eggs
- 250g ramen noodles
- 2 large handfuls shredded spring greens
- 4 spring onions, finely chopped
- 75g bamboo shoots from a can, drained, chopped and soaked in 2 tbsp rice vinegar
- pickled chilli and shallots (optional)
- chilli oil, to serve

FOR THE RAMEN STOCK
- 6 chicken legs
- 2 large carrots, halved
- 2 onions, quartered
- 4cm piece ginger, sliced
- 4 dried shiitake mushrooms
- 900g piece pork shoulder (thick layer of fat removed), halved

FOR THE RAMEN SEASONING
- 1 tbsp mirin
- 1 tbsp saké
- 4 tbsp Japanese soy sauce

1 Heat oven to 200C/180C fan/gas 6. For the stock, put the chicken, carrots, onions and ginger in a large roasting tin. Sprinkle with seasoning and roast for 30 mins. Transfer everything from the tin, including the fat and juices, to a large saucepan. Add the shiitake mushrooms and the pork, and pour in 3 litres of cold water. Bring to the boil and turn down to the lowest simmer you can. After the foamy scum rises to the top, skim it off with a ladle and discard. Part-cover with a lid. Let it simmer for 3 hrs but remove the pork after about 2½ hrs, or when it is very soft, and set aside. Strain the stock into a clean pan. Save the chicken and use it for something else. Boil for another 30–40 mins on a medium heat to reduce by a third, then skim the excess fat off. Add about 1 tsp salt and taste to see if it needs more.
2 Boil the eggs in a pan for 6 mins, then remove and put in iced water to cool.
3 Boil the noodles in a large pan, stirring so they don't stick, until al dente, about 3 mins. In the final minute of cooking, add the greens. Drain and divide among the bowls.
4 Mix the ramen seasoning ingredients in a small bowl. Slice the pork and add to the bowls. Pour the broth over each and add the spring onions and bamboo shoots. Peel the eggs, slice in half lengthways and place in each bowl with a dollop of pickled chilli and shallots, if you like. Pass round the ramen seasoning and chilli oil to serve on top.

Nutrition: *per serving*
kcal 798 fat 32g saturates 10g carbs 51g sugars 4g fibre 4g protein 71g salt 6g

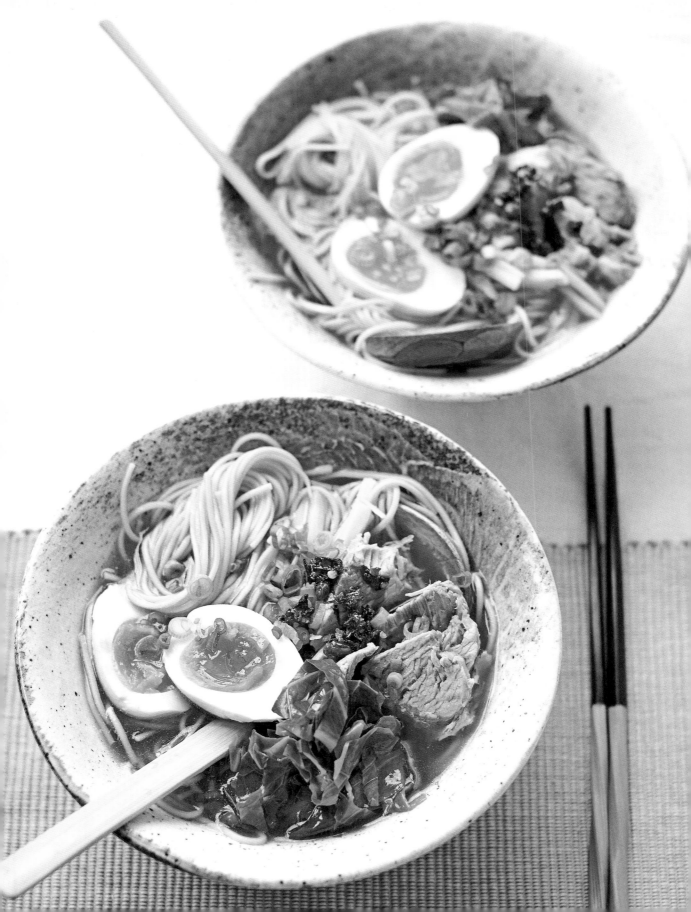

Beef goulash soup

Caraway seeds add an aromatic aniseed note to this soup. You could replace them with fennel seeds, for a similar flavour.

🕐 PREP 15 mins COOK 1 hr 🥧 3

- 1 tbsp extra virgin rapeseed oil
- 1 large onion, halved and sliced
- 3 garlic cloves, sliced
- 200g extra lean stewing beef, finely diced
- 1 tsp caraway seeds
- 2 tsp smoked paprika
- 400g can chopped tomatoes
- 600ml beef stock
- 1 medium sweet potato, peeled and diced
- 1 green pepper, deseeded and diced
- 150g pot natural bio yogurt
- good handful parsley, chopped

1 Heat the oil in a large pan, add the onion and garlic, and fry for 5 mins until starting to colour. Stir in the beef, increase the heat and fry, stirring, to brown it.
2 Add the caraway and paprika, stir well, then tip in the tomatoes and stock. Cover and leave to cook gently for 30 mins.
3 Stir in the sweet potato and green pepper, cover and cook for 20 mins more or until tender. Allow to cool a little, then serve topped with the yogurt and parsley (if the soup is too hot, it will kill the beneficial bacteria in the yogurt).

Nutrition: *per serving*
kcal 345 fat 12g saturates 4g carbs 28g sugars 18g fibre 7g protein 25g salt 1g

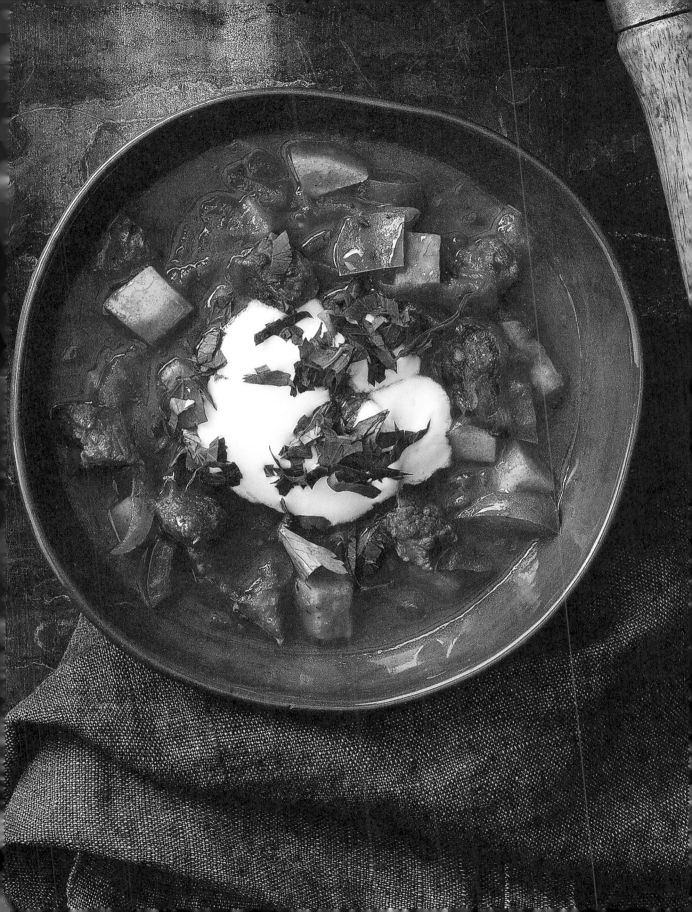

Kadala curry

Chickpeas are high in protein, and therefore perfect if you're vegetarian. This recipe is loaded with lots of other superfood ingredients, such as the warming spices.

🕐 PREP 15 mins COOK 25 mins 🥧 4

FOR THE PASTE
- 2 tbsp oil
- 1 onion, diced
- 1 tsp fresh or dried chilli, to taste
- 9 garlic cloves (approx 1 small bulb of garlic)
- thumb-sized piece ginger, peeled
- 1 tbsp ground coriander
- 2 tbsp ground cumin
- 1 tbsp garam masala
- 2 tbsp tomato purée

FOR THE CURRY
- 2 x 400g cans chickpeas, drained
- 400g can chopped tomatoes
- 100g creamed coconut
- ½ small pack coriander, chopped, plus extra to garnish
- 100g spinach
- cooked brown rice, to serve

1 To make the paste, heat a little of the oil in a frying pan, add the onion and chilli, and cook until softened, about 8 mins. Meanwhile, in a food processor, combine the garlic, ginger and remaining oil, then add the spices, tomato purée, ½ tsp salt and the fried onion and chilli. Blend to a smooth paste – add a drop of water or more oil, if needed.

2 Cook the paste in a medium saucepan for 2 mins over a medium-high heat, stirring occasionally so it doesn't stick. Tip in the chickpeas and chopped tomatoes, and simmer for 5 mins until reduced down. Add the coconut with a little water, cook for 5 mins more, then add the coriander and spinach, and cook until wilted. Garnish with extra coriander and serve with rice.

Nutrition: *per serving*
kcal 458 fat 28g saturates 16g carbs 31g sugars 9g fibre 10g protein 15g salt 0.2g

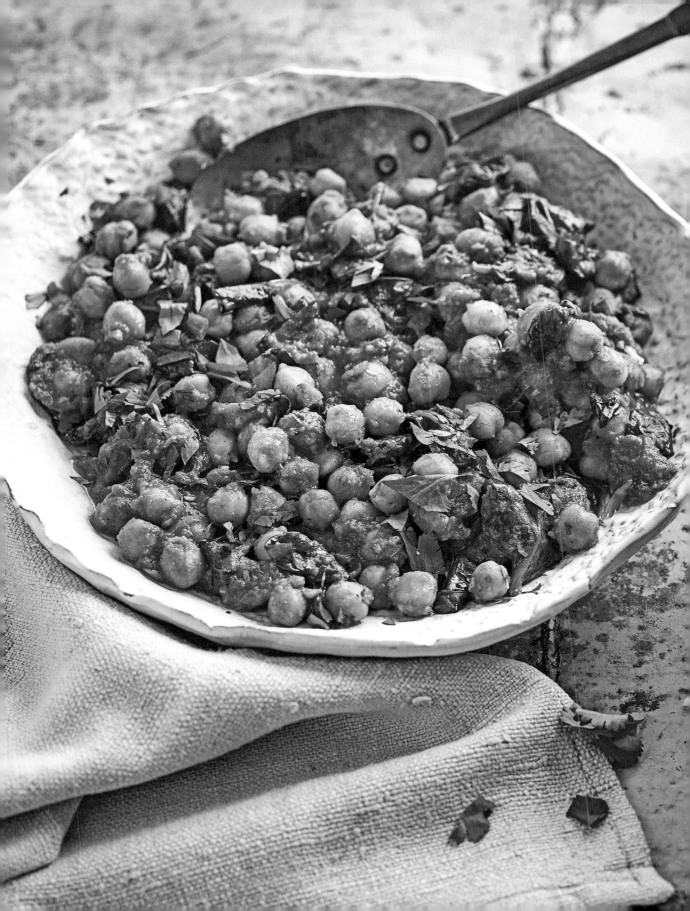

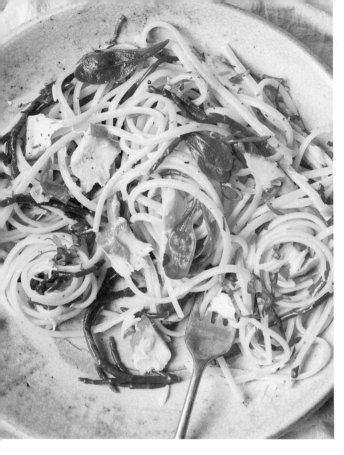

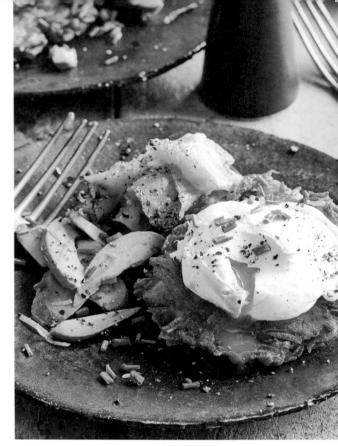

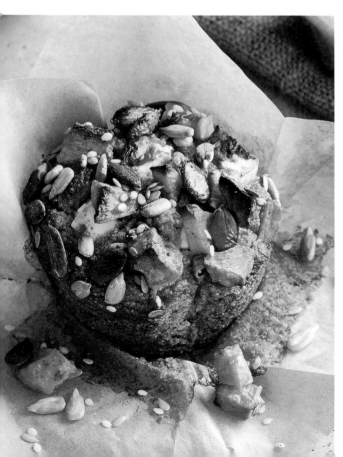

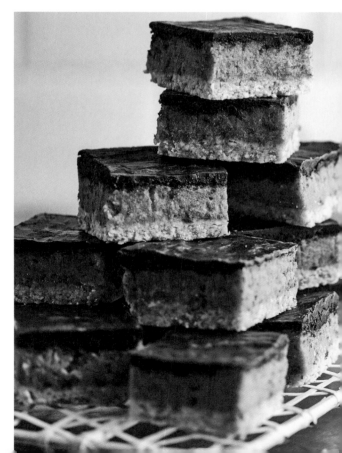

Chapter 2:

FABULOUS FATS

· ·

Fat adds flavour to a dish and is an essential component of a balanced, superfood diet. We need fat for healthy, supple skin, to lift our mood, improve concentration and focus as well as for a well-functioning immune system. Take that oil dressing on your salad, it plays an important role enhancing your absorption of fat-soluble vitamins (A, D, E and K), all vital for a healthy immune system.

A certain type of poly-unsaturated fat, known as omega-3 fatty acids, are found in their most potent form in oily species of fish like sardines, salmon and mackerel. These omega-3 fats are essential to health – we need them for a healthy heart and brain as well as balanced hormones. Experts tell us that we should eat at least one portion of these oily fish each week in order to meet our omega-3 needs. If your budget allows choose wild rather than farmed fish because of its superior fat content.

Plant sources of these beneficial omega-3 fats include walnuts, flaxseed and chia seeds.

Despite being a saturate you can enjoy butter in moderation as well as plant-based sat fats like coconut oil. Coconut oil is rich in medium-chain triglycerides, which are healthier for you because the liver burns them as energy, rather than storing them as fat. What's more, being a saturate, coconut oil is stable at high temperatures making it an ideal choice for roasting and frying.

We've packed our Key lime pie (page 70) and Made-over millionaire bars (page 72) full of healthy, superfood fats but don't forget all things in moderation! Fat is densely calorific, supplying 9 calories per gram rather than 4 calories per gram for carbs and protein – so *portion* size really does matter!

Masala frittata with avocado salsa

Not only are avocados a great source of healthy fats, they also provide vitamins E, B-vitamins, potassium and fibre.

PREP 15 mins COOK 25 mins 4

- 2 tbsp extra virgin rapeseed oil
- 3 onions, 2½ thinly sliced, ½ finely chopped
- 1 tbsp Madras curry paste
- 500g cherry tomatoes, halved
- 1 red chilli, deseeded and finely chopped
- small pack coriander, roughly chopped
- 8 large eggs, beaten
- 1 avocado, stoned, peeled and cubed
- juice 1 lemon

1 Heat the oil in a medium non-stick, ovenproof frying pan. Tip in the sliced onions and cook over a medium heat for about 10 mins until soft and golden. Add the Madras paste and fry for 1 min more, then tip in half the tomatoes and half the chilli. Cook until the mixture is thick and the tomatoes have all burst.

2 Heat the grill to high. Add half the coriander to the eggs and season, then pour over the spicy onion mixture. Stir gently once or twice, then cook over a low heat for 8–10 mins until almost set. Transfer to the grill for 3–5 mins until set.

3 To make the salsa, mix the avocado, remaining chilli and tomatoes, chopped onion, remaining coriander and the lemon juice together, then season and serve with the frittata.

Nutrition: *per serving*
kcal 347 fat 25g saturates 5g carbs 12g sugars 9g fibre 5g protein 16g salt 0.5g

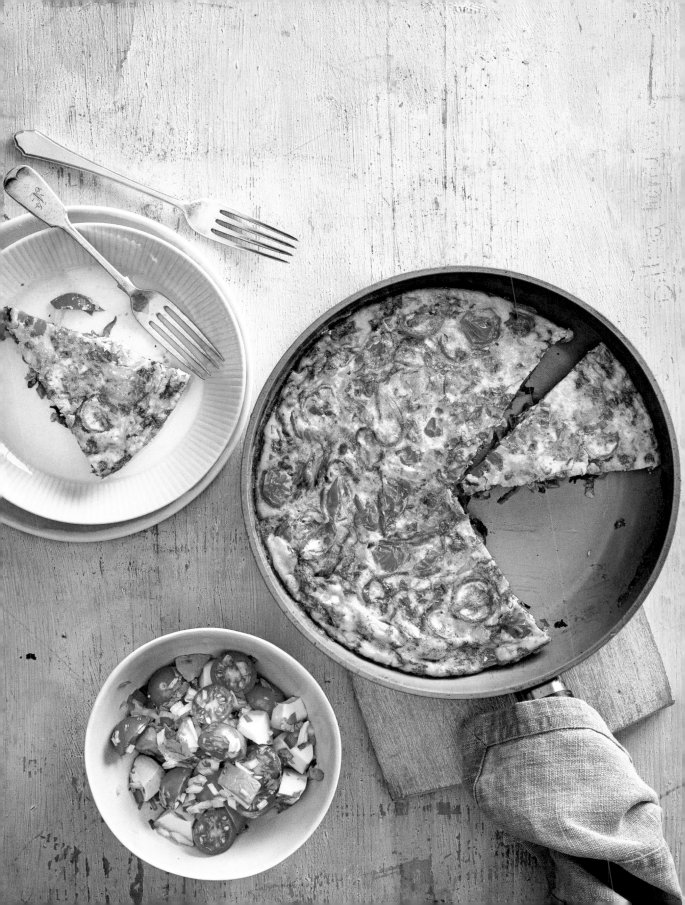

Samphire & lemony salmon linguine

Samphire is a sea vegetable, high in many nutrients, with a salty, fresh flavour. You can also use sea purslane (another nutrient-packed sea vegetable), asparagus or peas.

PREP 10 mins COOK 15 mins 2

- 2 tbsp olive oil
- ½ small preserved lemon, flesh and pith scooped out, skin finely chopped
- 2 large shallots, finely chopped
- ½ red chilli, finely sliced
- 1 tbsp finely chopped parsley stalks (reserve the leaves, to serve)
- small glass of rosé wine or white wine
- 175g linguine
- 80g samphire
- 100g cooked salmon, flaked into large pieces
- juice ½ lemon

1 Heat the olive oil in a heavy-bottomed, non-stick frying pan or skillet. Add the preserved lemon, shallot, chilli, parsley stalks and seasoning, and sweat for about 5 mins or until soft and fragrant. Pour in the wine and bubble for 1–2 mins.

2 Meanwhile, bring a large pot of salted water to the boil. Add the linguine and cook following pack instructions until just al dente. Throw the samphire into the water with the linguine. Cook for 30 secs, then drain everything, reserving a few ladlefuls of the pasta water.

3 Add the linguine and samphire to the frying pan with half a ladle of the pasta water. Add the salmon and lemon juice, and stir thoroughly to combine into a sauce, adding a splash more of the water if needed. Season to taste. Divide between plates and grind over some extra black pepper. Garnish with more chopped parsley, if you like

Nutrition: *per serving*
kcal 554 fat 23g saturates 4g carbs 52g sugars 5g fibre 5g protein 23g salt 1.3g

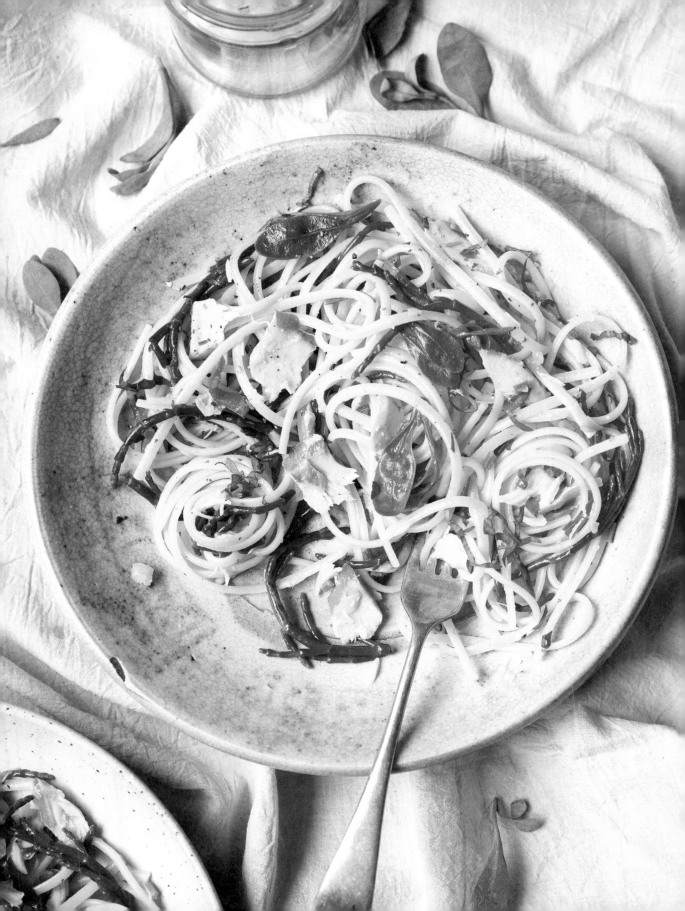

Scandi salmon salad

Improve your heart and brain health with this omega-3 packed dish.

PREP 15 mins COOK 30 mins 2

- 400g baby new potatoes halved
- 1 lemon
- 2 salmon fillets
- 150ml crème fraîche
- ½ pack dill, finely chopped
- ½ pack flat-leaf parsley, finely chopped
- 1 tbsp Dijon mustard
- ½ red onion, finely chopped
- 100g radishes quartered

1 Heat oven to 200C/180C fan/gas 6. Boil the potatoes in a large pan of salted water. Bring to the boil and cook for 15 mins, or until tender. Drain and set aside to cool.

2 Meanwhile, zest the lemon, set the zest aside and thinly slice half the lemon. Put the salmon on a baking sheet, season and top with the lemon slices. Roast in the oven for 12–15 mins, until just cooked through. Leave to cool.

3 Mix together the crème fraîche, dill, parsley, mustard, the reserved lemon zest and one squeeze of the remaining lemon half. Toss together the cooled potatoes with the onion, radish and dressing. Flake over the salmon and season.

Nutrition: *per serving*
kcal 694 fat 43g saturates 23g carbs 40g sugars 7g fibre 4g protein 32g salt 1g

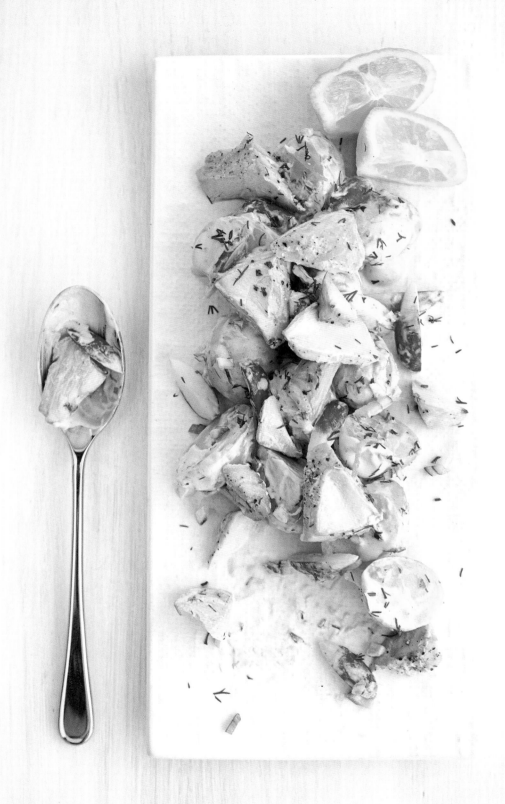

Horseradish latkes with avocado, gravadlax & poached eggs

This dish has a double whammy of healthy fats with omega-3 rich salmon and avocados. It makes a great breakfast or light dinner.

PREP 15 mins COOK 15 mins 2

- 2 baking potatoes (about 500g), peeled
- 2 tbsp plain flour
- 3 very fresh large eggs
- 2 tsp creamed horseradish
- small bunch chives, snipped
- pinch of white pepper (or to taste)
- vegetable oil or sunflower oil
- 2 tbsp white wine vinegar
- 1 ripe avocado
- zest and juice ½ lemon
- 150g gravadlax or smoked salmon

1 Grate the potatoes on the coarse side of a box grater straight onto a clean tea towel. Gather the tea towel together and squeeze out as much liquid as you can from the potatoes. Tip the potatoes into a bowl and add the flour, 1 egg, the horseradish and most of the chives (reserve some to serve). Season with salt and white pepper – white pepper is hotter than black, so go easy. Mix well.

2 Heat the oven to its lowest setting, with a tray on one shelf. Heat the oil in a large frying pan – it should completely cover the base. Have a plate covered with kitchen paper ready. When the oil is hot, spoon mounds of the potato mixture into the pan – they should be about 10cm wide. Press them down with the back of a fish slice and cook for 3–4 mins each side, or until golden brown and crispy, and the potato is cooked through. Transfer them to the kitchen paper to drain off the excess oil, then keep warm on the tray while you continue cooking until all the mixture is used up (makes 6 latkes in total).

3 Heat a large pan of water until bubbles are just breaking the surface but it's not rapidly boiling, then add the vinegar. Crack an egg into a small bowl, then drop the egg into the pan. Do the same with the remaining egg, cook for 2–3 mins until poached to your liking, then scoop out in the same order you dropped them in and drain on kitchen paper. Halve and stone the avocado, then ease a dessertspoon between the skin and the flesh to remove each half. Slice the avocado, then squeeze over the lemon juice.

4 To serve, arrange the latkes over 2 plates, and top with the gravadlax, avocado and poached eggs. Scatter with the remaining chives, the lemon zest and a little black pepper, if you like.

Nutrition: *per serving*
kcal 796 fat 38g saturates 7g carbs 72g sugars 5g fibre 10g protein 37g salt 2.6g

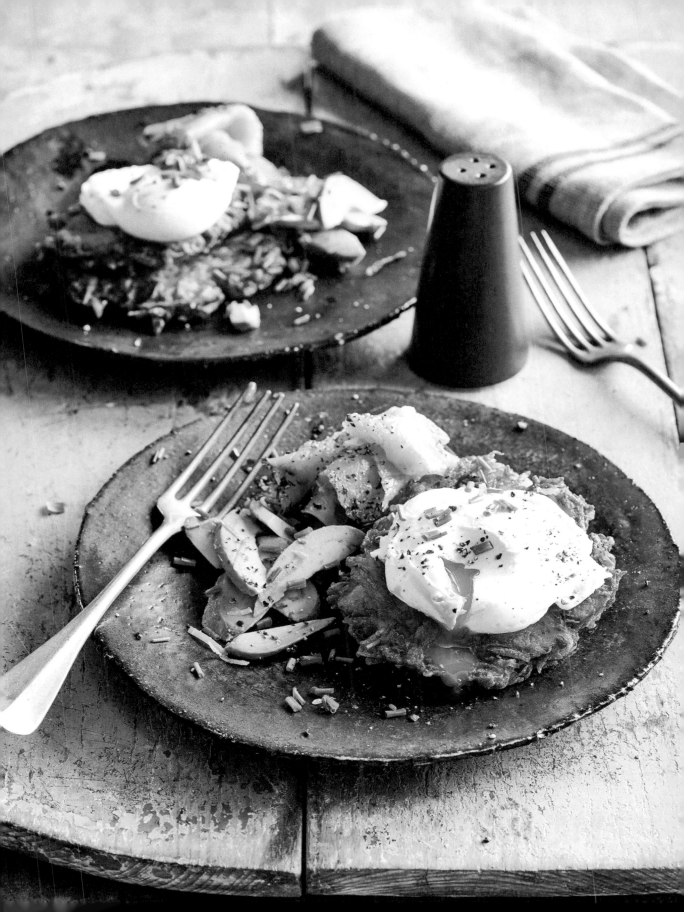

Open rye sandwich with chicken & avocado

· ·

This speedy lunch recipe will be on the table in just 5 mins. Use a fresh variety of guacamole, or make your own by mashing avocado, lime juice and coriander.

🕐 PREP 5 mins NO COOK 🥧 2

- 2 tbsp guacamole
- 2 slices rye bread
- 8 slices tomato
- 2 cooked chicken breasts, sliced, we used Cajun spiced chicken
- squeeze of lime

1 Divide guacamole between rye bread, spreading it evenly. Arrange 4 slices of tomato on each sandwich, and top with a sliced chicken breast. Finish with lime juice and some ground black pepper.

· ·

Nutrition: *per serving*
kcal 327 fat 10g saturates 2g carbs 27g sugars 5g fibre 9g protein 27g salt 0.9g

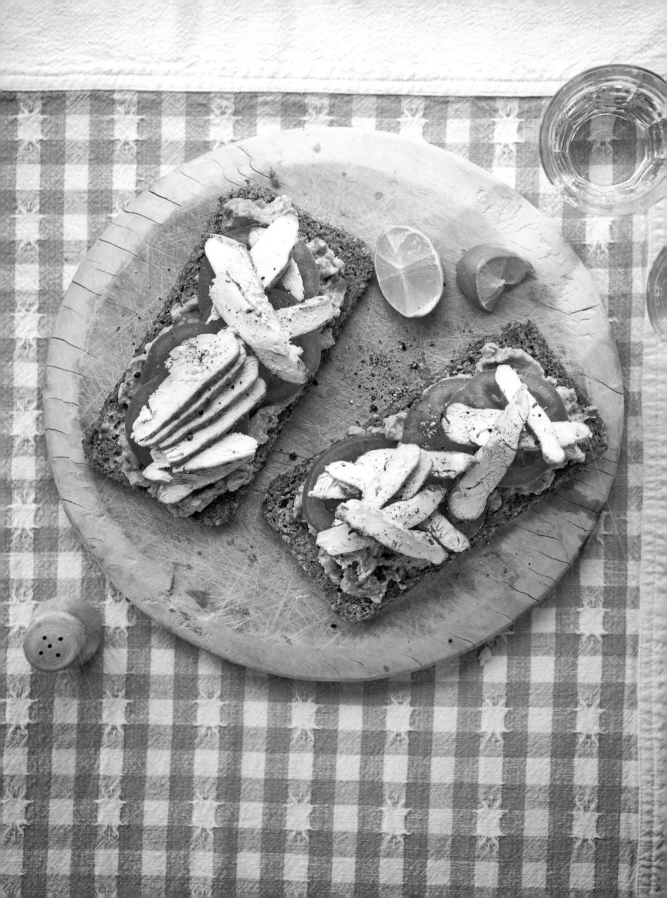

Marinated mackerel with green olive & celery dressing

Mackerel is best when it's very fresh. Look out for bright eyes and firm flesh when buying mackerel, and don't forget to give it a sniff – it should smell of the sea, fresh but not fishy.

PREP 10 mins COOK plus chilling and marinating 4

- 2 mackerel, filleted and pin bones removed
- ½ tsp fennel seeds, toasted
- 150ml olive oil
- 3 banana shallots, sliced into rings
- 1½ tbsp golden caster sugar
- juice ½ lemon
- 150ml red wine vinegar
- 10 green olives, pitted and halved
- 2 celery sticks, thinly sliced at an angle
- 1 tsp chopped celery leaves
- lemon wedges, to serve
- crème fraîche, to serve (optional)

1 Lay the mackerel fillets, skin-side down, in a shallow dish, then sprinkle with the fennel seeds and 1½ tbsp flaky salt, making sure you cover the fish evenly. Cover with cling film and put in the fridge for 1 hr, then remove, wash off the salt and fennel seeds, and pat the fish dry with kitchen paper.

2 Return the fish to the shallow dish, skin-side up, pour over the olive oil and scatter over the shallots. Put the sugar, lemon juice and vinegar in a small saucepan and bring to the boil, then pour the hot liquid over the fish. Leave to cool, cover in cling film and put in the fridge to marinate overnight.

3 The next day, remove the fish from the fridge 1 hr before serving to bring it to room temperature, then transfer to a serving plate. Stir in the olives, celery and celery leaves. Leave for a few mins, then serve with lemon wedges and a couple of spoonfuls of crème fraîche.

Nutrition: *per serving*
kcal 638 fat 58g saturates 10g carbs 8g sugars 8g fibre 1g protein 20g salt 1.8g

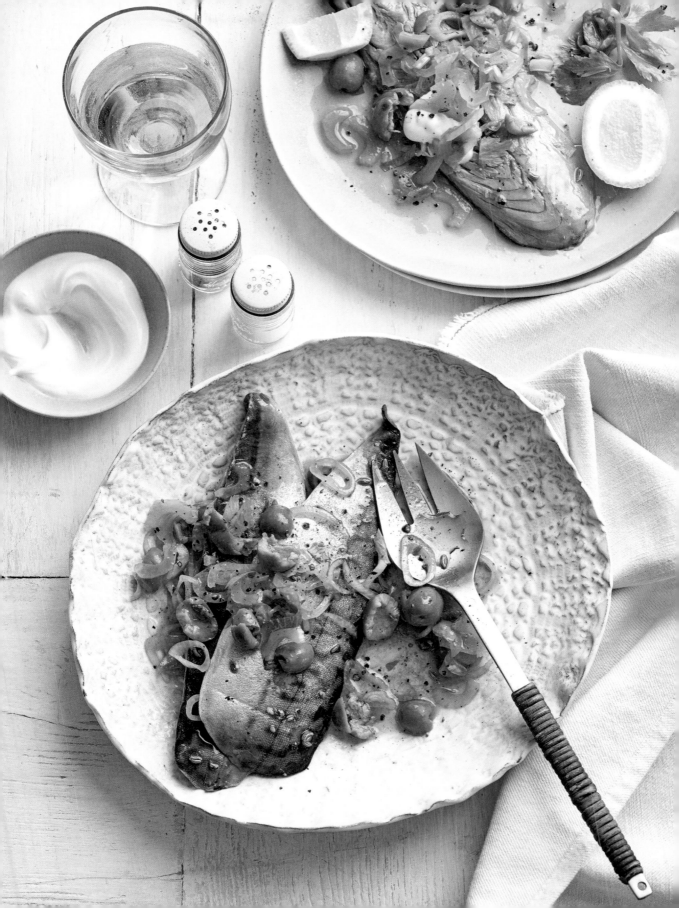

California avocado & quinoa salad

This colourful salad will give you a lunchbox to be envied, take the dressing in a separate pot to drizzle over just before eating.

🕐 PREP 10 mins COOK 30 mins 🥧 2

- 250g butternut squash, chopped into small chunks
- 2 tbsp olive oil or extra virgin rapeseed oil
- 120g pack thin-stemmed broccoli, cut into small pieces
- 250g pouch cooked quinoa
- small handful coriander, leaves picked and chopped
- small handful mint, leaves picked and chopped
- 4 spring onions, finely sliced on an angle
- 50g pomegranate seeds
- 20g pistachios, roughly chopped
- 1 small ripe avocado
- juice ½ lemon
- handful sprouts (alfalfa or china rose sprouts are nice) or baby herb leaves

FOR THE DRESSING
- 1 tbsp tahini
- ½ small ripe avocado, stoned, peeled and roughly chopped
- small handful coriander, leaves picked
- small handful mint, leaves picked
- zest and juice ½ lemon
- 2 tsp clear honey or maple syrup

1 Heat oven to 200C/180C fan/gas 6 and line a baking tray with parchment. Tip the butternut squash onto the tray, drizzle with 2 tsp oil and season well. Roast for 20 mins, then push the squash to one end of the tray, add the broccoli to the other end and drizzle with 1 tsp oil. Season and roast for 10 mins more.
2 Meanwhile, make the dressing. Put all the ingredients in the small bowl of a food processor, add 1 tbsp water and a pinch of salt. Blitz to make a loose dressing, adding a little more water if necessary.
3 Squeeze the pouch of quinoa to separate the grains, then tip into a large bowl. Add the herbs, spring onions, pomegranate seeds and pistachios. Add the remaining 1 tbsp oil, season and toss everything together. Add the roasted veg too.
4 Divide the salad between two plates and drizzle over the dressing. Halve the avocado and remove the stone, then slide a dessertspoon between the skin and flesh to remove it in one piece. Place on a chopping board, rounded side up, and thinly slice. Squeeze over the lemon juice, then slide a knife underneath and lift half the avocado onto each salad. Top with the sprouts and grind over a little pepper, if you like.

Nutrition: *per serving*
kcal 740 fat 44g saturates 6g carbs 59g sugars 17g fibre 17g protein 18g salt 0.9g

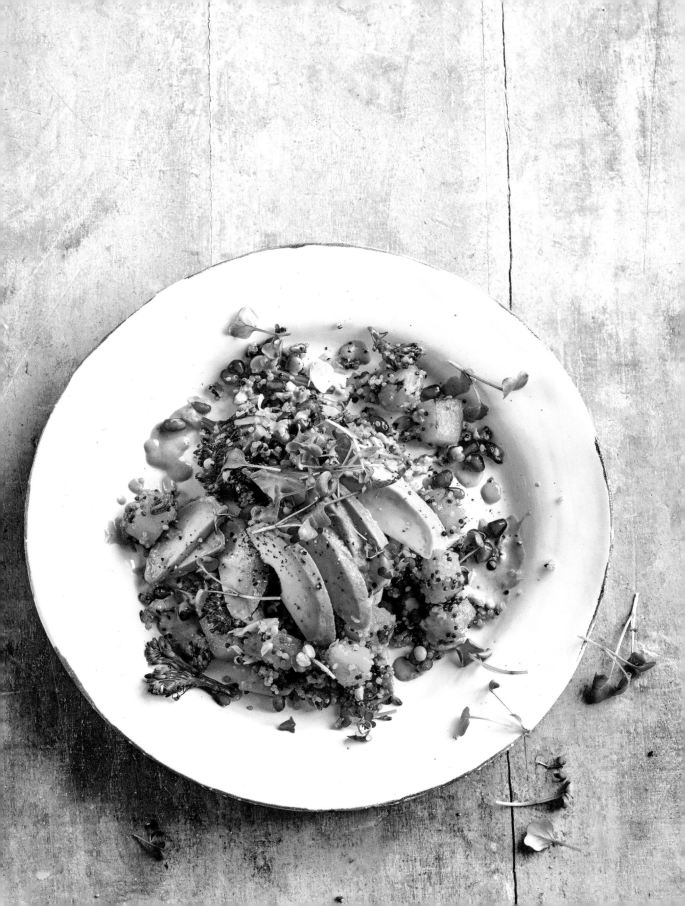

Smoked mackerel maki rolls

This is a nice recipe to make with kids, and if they haven't tried mackerel before it will encourage them to give it a go.

PREP 20 mins COOK 25 mins 4

- 150g sushi rice
- 2 tsp rice wine vinegar
- 4 nori sheets
- 1 red chilli, deseeded and cut into matchsticks
- ½ carrot, peeled and cut into matchsticks
- ¼ cucumber, cut into matchsticks
- 100g smoked mackerel, skin removed, torn into small pieces
- soy sauce, for dipping

1 Put the rice in a small bowl, cover with cold water and massage the grains with your hands to remove the starch. Drain and repeat the process until the water runs clear.

2 Put the rice in a small saucepan with a tight-fitting lid. Cover with 2.5cm of cold water, put the lid on and simmer over a medium heat for 10 mins. Take off the heat and leave with the lid on for a further 15 mins. Stir through the vinegar, then leave to cool completely.

3 Fill a small bowl with cold water and lay out a sushi mat. Place a nori sheet, shiny-side down, on top of the sushi mat. Spread a quarter of the rice onto the nori, leaving a 1cm border at the top.

4 Put a quarter of the chilli and carrot in a line at the bottom of the rice. Place a quarter of the cucumber and mackerel in a strip along the centre. Dampen the top border with a little water to help seal the roll. Fold the bottom edge of the seaweed over the first line of the filling, then use the sushi mat to roll up the maki. Repeat to make four rolls. Using a serrated knife, cut each roll into eight rounds. Serve with soy sauce for dipping.

Nutrition: *per serving*
kcal 218 fat 6g saturates 1g carbs 30g sugars 2g fibre 3g protein 9g salt 0.6g

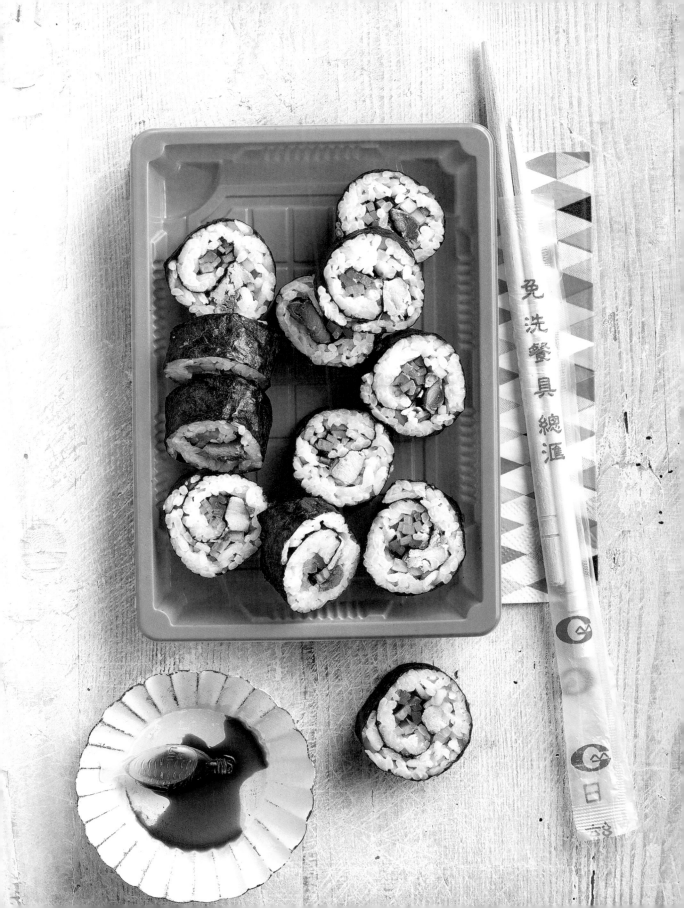

Sweet potato, avocado & feta muffins

We've used creamy avocado to replace some of the fat in these healthy savoury muffins. Eat them as a snack, or with soup for lunch.

PREP 20 mins COOK 30 mins 9

- 1 sweet potato (about 200g), peeled and chopped into small chunks
- drizzle of flavourless oil, such as vegetable or sunflower
- 1 large avocado, peel and stone removed, roughly chopped (about 150g prepared weight)
- 100g ground almonds
- 100g fine polenta
- 80ml maple syrup
- 3 large eggs
- 1½ tsp baking powder
- 1 tsp bicarbonate of soda
- 100ml whole milk
- 50g feta, crumbled (optional)
- 2 tbsp mixed seeds
- ¼ tsp sweet paprika

1 Place the sweet potato in a heatproof bowl, cover with cling film and microwave on High for 8 mins, or until really soft. Leave to cool completely. Grease 9 holes of a muffin tin with a little oil (or line each hole with a square of baking parchment.)

2 Chop ¼ of the sweet potato into even smaller pieces and set aside. Place the remaining sweet potato, avocado, almonds, polenta, maple syrup, eggs, baking powder, bicarb, milk and ¼ tsp salt in the bowl of a food processor. Blend until completely smooth. Divide the mixture evenly among the muffin tin holes, then top with the reserved chopped sweet potato, feta, seeds and a dusting of paprika. Bake for 22 mins at 180C/160 fan/ gas mark 4, or until risen, browning on top and cooked through – check by inserting a skewer to the centre, it should come out dry. Cool in the tin for 5 mins, then transfer to a wire rack and cool completely. Store in a sealed container for up to 3 days.

Nutrition: *per muffin*
kcal 275 fat 16g saturates 3g carbs 22g sugars 10g fibre 3g protein 9g salt 0.9g

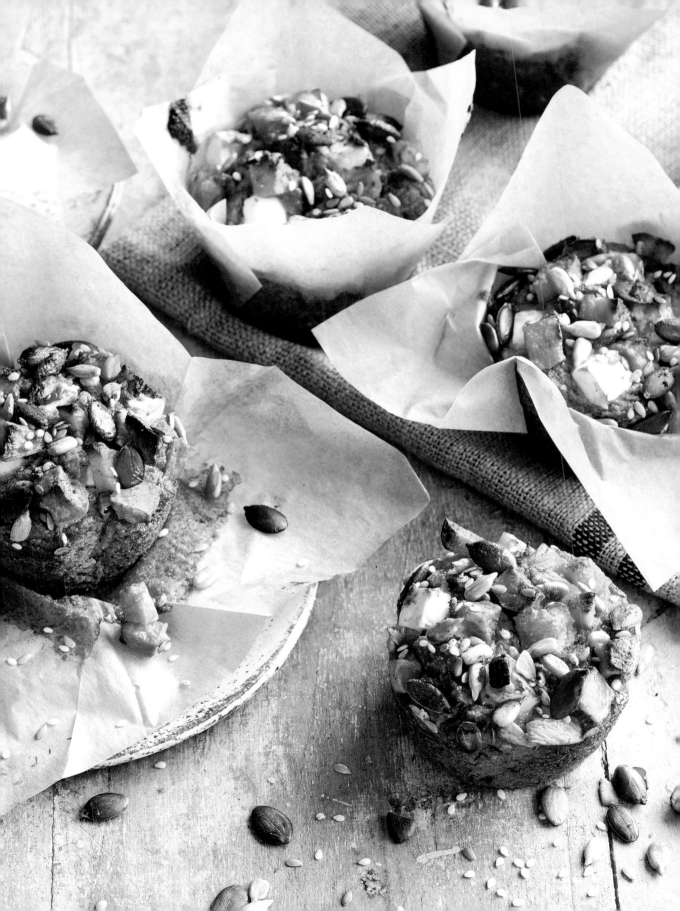

Curried aubergine with bavette

Coconut cream adds a lovely flavour and rich texture to this curry, it also contains healthy medium-chain triglycerides.

PREP 10 mins COOK 25 mins 4

- 2 tbsp vegetable oil, plus a drizzle
- 2 banana shallots, thinly sliced
- 2 garlic cloves, finely chopped
- 2 tsp coriander seeds
- 2 tsp cumin seeds
- 1 tsp turmeric
- 2 tsp garam masala
- 2 aubergines, cut into small cubes
- 60g creamed coconut
- 2 naan breads
- 10g butter
- 300g bavette steak
- 50g flaked almonds, toasted
- 50g pomegranate seeds
- natural yogurt and mango chutney, to serve (optional)

1 Heat the oil in a sauté pan with a lid over a medium heat. Add the shallots and cook for 8 mins, stirring occasionally, until softened. Stir in the garlic and cook for 1 min more, then add the spices. Cook for a further 30 secs until fragrant.

2 Tip in the aubergine and give everything a good stir to coat in the spice mix. Add the creamed coconut, a pinch of salt and 500ml boiling water. Break down the creamed coconut with the back of a wooden spoon, then put the lid on and cook for 15 mins until the aubergine is tender.

3 Meanwhile, heat oven to 180C/160C fan/gas 4. Dot the butter over the naans, then put them on a large baking tray to warm through for 5 mins. Heat a drizzle of oil in a pan and cook the bavette to your liking, 2–3 mins per side for medium rare, or longer if you prefer it more well done. Tear the naans into pieces and slice the steak.

4 Taste the aubergine for seasoning, then pile up the bavette in the middle of the curry. Sprinkle over the almonds, pomegranate seeds, and a dollop of yogurt and mango chutney, if using. Serve from the pan in the middle of the table with the naan on the side for scooping.

Nutrition: *per serving*
kcal 630 fat 41g saturates 16g carbs 29g sugars 10g fibre 8g protein 32g salt 0.5g

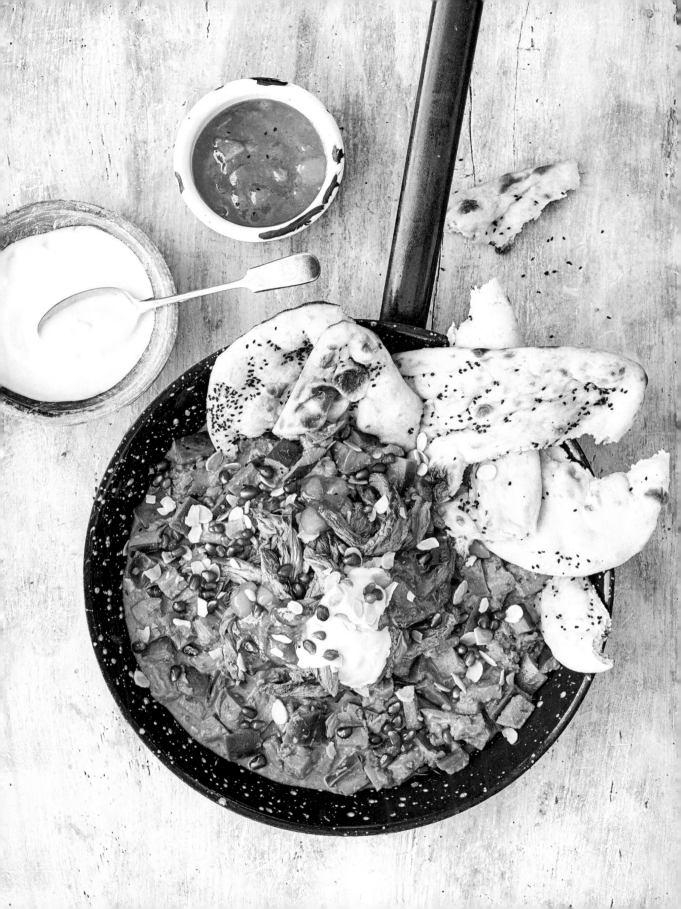

Fish mappas

A coconut fish curry, popular in the southern Indian state of Kerala – use pollock or any other sustainably sourced white fish fillets

PREP 15 mins COOK 20 mins 4

- 300g basmati rice
- 1 tbsp sunflower or vegetable oil
- 2 large onions, sliced
- 2 garlic cloves, chopped
- 450g tomatoes, cut into chunks
- 3 tbsp tikka curry paste
- 400g can coconut milk
- 4 skinless, boneless pollock fillets (about 150g each), or other sustainable white fish, cut into 4cm chunks
- ½ small pack coriander, roughly chopped

1 Put a large saucepan of water on to boil and cook the rice following pack instructions. Meanwhile, heat the oil in a large, wide saucepan over a medium heat and add the onions. Cook for 5–10 mins until softened and starting to colour. Add the garlic and tomatoes, and fry for 2 mins. Add the curry paste, fry for 2 mins more, then pour in the coconut milk and bring to the boil.

2 Add the fish to the pan and simmer gently for 5–8 mins until just cooked through. Turn off the heat. Sprinkle the coriander over the curry and serve with the rice.

Nutrition: per serving
kcal 691 fat 26g saturates 16g carbs 74g sugars 11g fibre 4g protein 39g salt 0.8g

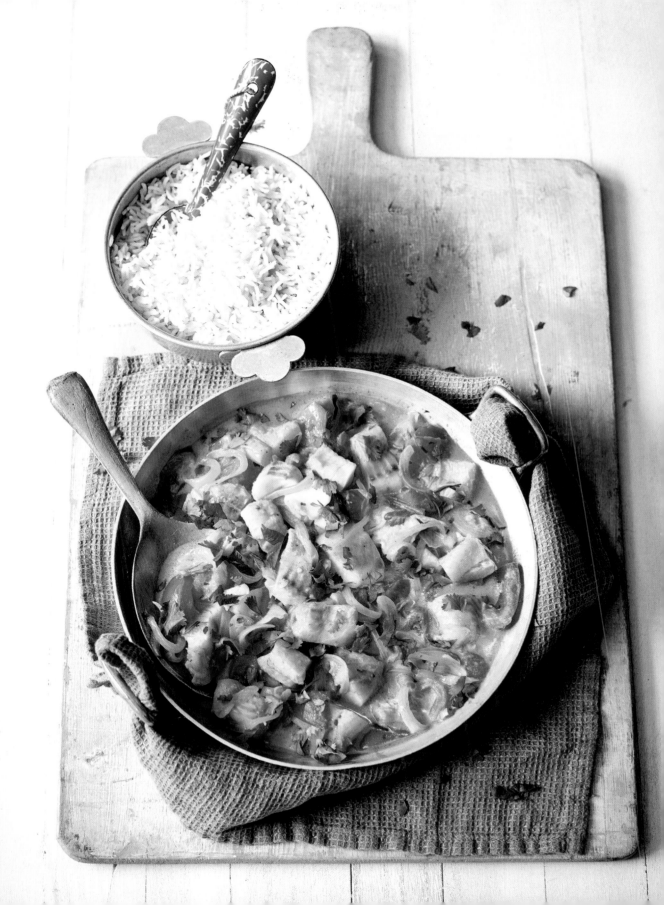

Sardines & tomatoes on toast

Tinned sardines are a cost-effective way to get plenty of heart-healthy oily fish. Keep a can in the cupboard for a quick dinner or lunch for one

PREP 10 mins NO COOK 1

- 2 slices sourdough bread, toasted
- 1 large garlic clove, halved
- 135g can sardines in olive oil
- 130g cherry tomatoes, halved
- handful watercress
- 1 tbsp parsley, roughly chopped
- ½ lemon, to serve (optional)

1 Rub each piece of toast with the garlic. In a small bowl, mix the sardines and their oil with the tomatoes and the watercress, then season. Sit half the mixture on each slice of toast, piled high. Scatter over the parsley and squeeze over the lemon, if you like.

Nutrition: *per serving*
kcal 444 fat 16g saturates 4g carbs 39g sugars 7g fibre 4g protein 33g salt 2.1g

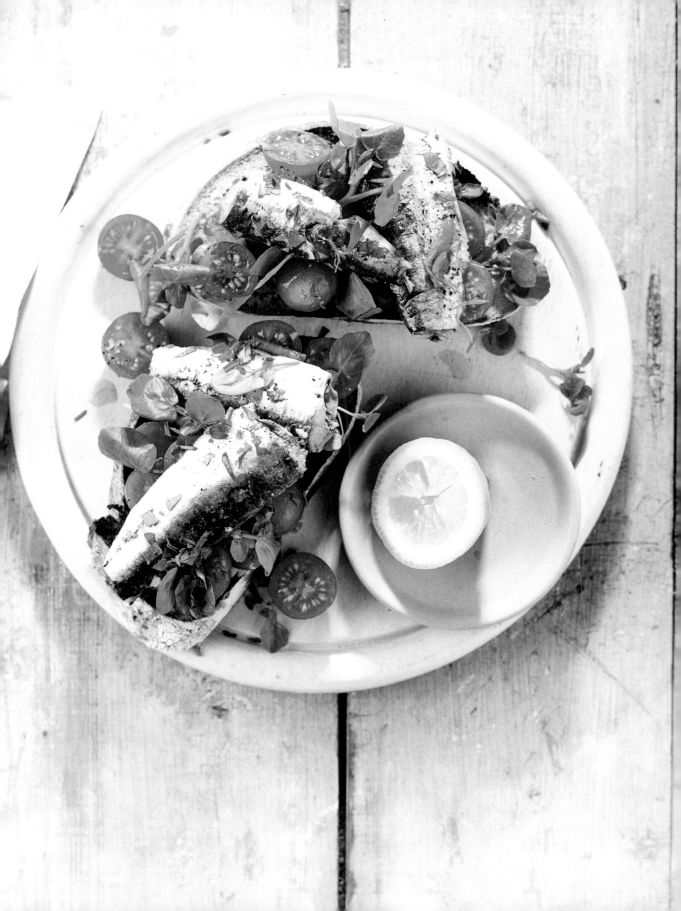

Chocolate, avocado & peanut butter pudding

Avocado's neutral flavour and creamy texture makes it a wonderful substitute for dairy in desserts or smoothies. These little pots will keep for a few days in the fridge – a great make-ahead dessert!

PREP 10 mins plus chilling NO COOK ⏲ 4

- 2 large, ripe avocados, halved and stoned
- 1 large banana, chopped
- 5 soft prunes
- 6 tbsp unsweetened almond milk or coconut milk
- 2 tbsp smooth peanut butter (unsweetened, if possible)
- 3 tbsp cacao powder (or good quality cocoa powder)
- 100g coconut milk yogurt (such as CoYo)
- 2 tsp maple syrup or honey
- dark chocolate (80% cocoa, if possible), to decorate

1 Scoop the avocado flesh into a food processor. Add the chopped banana, prunes, almond or coconut milk, smooth peanut butter and cacao powder. Blend until smooth, adding a little more milk if the blade gets stuck. Scrape down the sides once or twice and blend again.

2 Divide the mixture among 4 small glasses. Mix the coconut yogurt with the maple syrup or honey and top each pudding with a generous dollop. Finely grate a little dark chocolate over the top and chill for at least 1 hr.

Nutrition: *per serving*
kcal 394 fat 30g saturates 10g carbs 19g sugars 14g fibre 8g protein 6g salt 0.1g

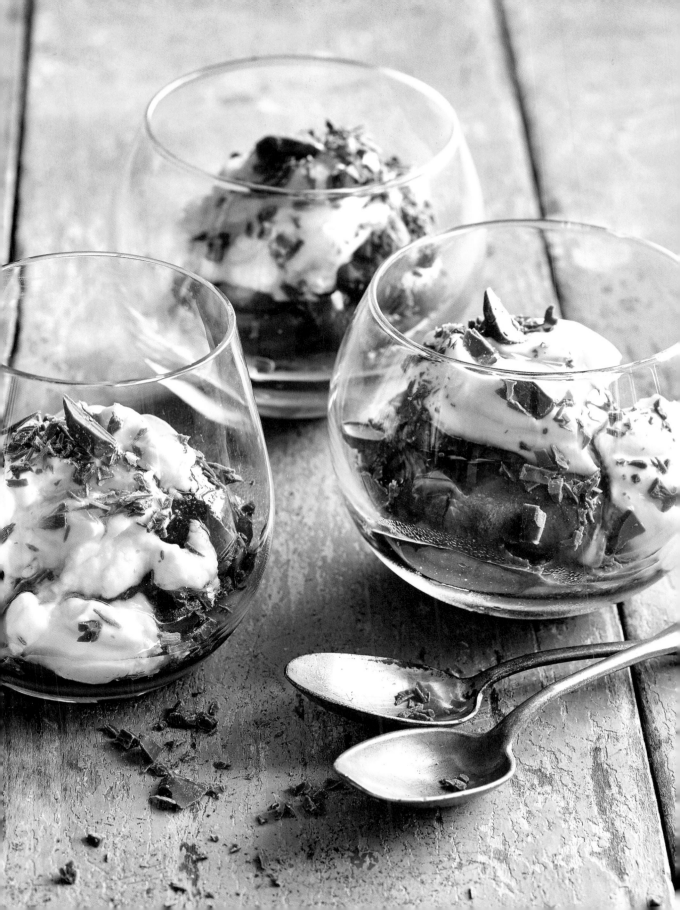

Key lime pie

This creamy, dairy-free (if you leave out the cream) dessert is naturally sweetened and uses entirely raw ingredients, with a date, walnut and coconut crust and a creamy avocado and cashew nut filling.

🕐 PREP 25 mins plus chilling NO COOK 🕐 12

- zest 1 lime, plus a few thin slices to decorate (optional)

FOR THE CRUST
- 225g pitted dates, soaked for 4–6 hrs if very dry
- 100g walnuts
- 45g desiccated coconut
- 30g cacao powder
- 1 tsp salt

FOR THE FILLING
- 200g cashew nuts, soaked for 4–6 hrs
- 240ml lime juice (juice of about 8 limes)
- 1½ ripe avocados
- ½ ripe mango
- 210g coconut oil, melted
- 110g agave nectar

1 Whizz all the crust ingredients in a food processor. Transfer the mixture to a 23cm loose-based tart tin. Using your fist, press the mixture evenly into the base and sides of the tin.
2 To prepare the filling, blend all the ingredients in a blender on a high-speed setting, until smooth and creamy.
3 Pour the filling onto the crust and shake the tin a little to even it out. Chill for a minimum of 3 hrs to set. Top with the lime zest and slices, if you like. Will keep in the freezer for up to 2 months. Defrosted in the fridge, it will keep for 1 week.

Nutrition: *per serving*
kcal 477 fat 38g saturates 20g carbs 26g sugars 22g fibre 5g protein 7g salt 0.4g

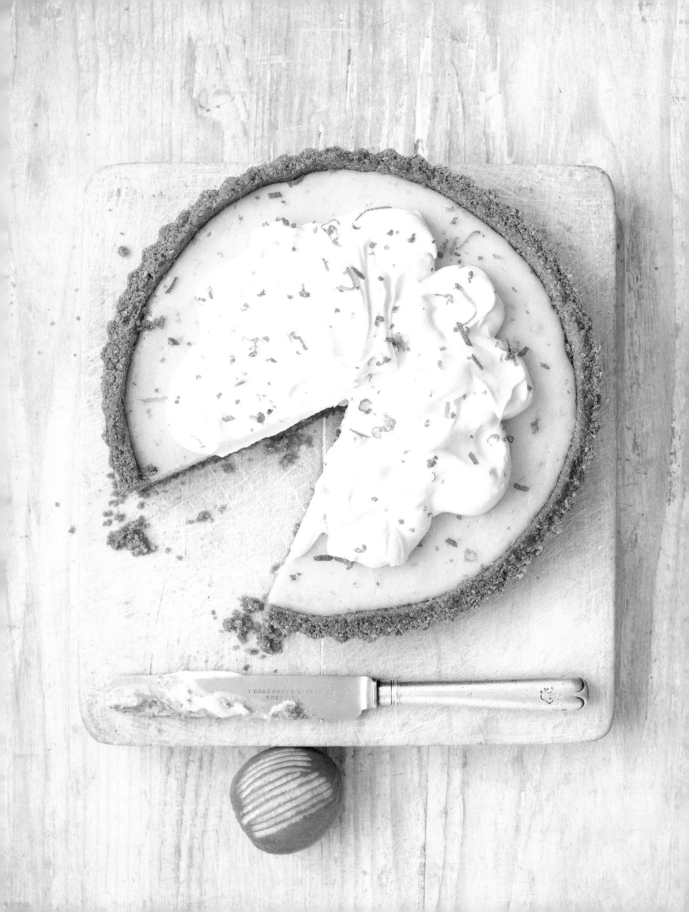

Made-over millionaire bars

These vegan, gluten-free chocolatey treats with dates, cashews and maple syrup are just as sticky and moreish as the original Millionaire's shortbreads.

PREP 30 mins COOK 5 mins plus chilling 16

FOR THE BASE
- 150g cashew nuts
- 50g rolled oat
- 4 Medjool dates, pitted
- 50g coconut oil, melted

FOR THE FILLING
- 350g pitted Medjool dates
- 125ml unsweetened almond milk
- 25ml maple syrup
- 150g coconut oil
- 1 tsp vanilla extract

FOR THE TOPPING
- 150g coconut oil
- 5 tbsp cocoa powder
- 2 tsp maple syrup

1 Grease a 20cm square cake tin and line with baking parchment. Tip the cashew nuts and oats into a food processer and blitz to crumbs. Add the dates and coconut oil, and blend again. Transfer to the tin and use a spoon to press the nutty mixture into a compact, even layer that covers the base. Chill while you prepare the filling.

2 For the filling, add the dates, almond milk, maple syrup and coconut oil to a saucepan with a generous pinch of salt and bring to a simmer. Boil for 2–3 mins until the dates are really soft, then tip into the blender, add the vanilla extract and blitz to a smooth purée. Add a little more salt if the mixture is too sweet. Pour over the nutty base and spread to the sides of the tin, getting the surface as smooth as possible. Chill while you prepare the topping.

3 Gently heat the coconut oil in a saucepan until melted. Remove from the heat and whisk in the cocoa and maple syrup until there are no lumps. Cool for 10 mins, pour over the caramel layer and return to the fridge for at least 3 hrs or until firmly set. To serve, cut into squares. Will keep in the fridge for up to 1 week.

Nutrition: *per square*
kcal 373 fat 28g saturates 20g carbs 25g sugars 20g fibre 3g protein 4g salt 0g

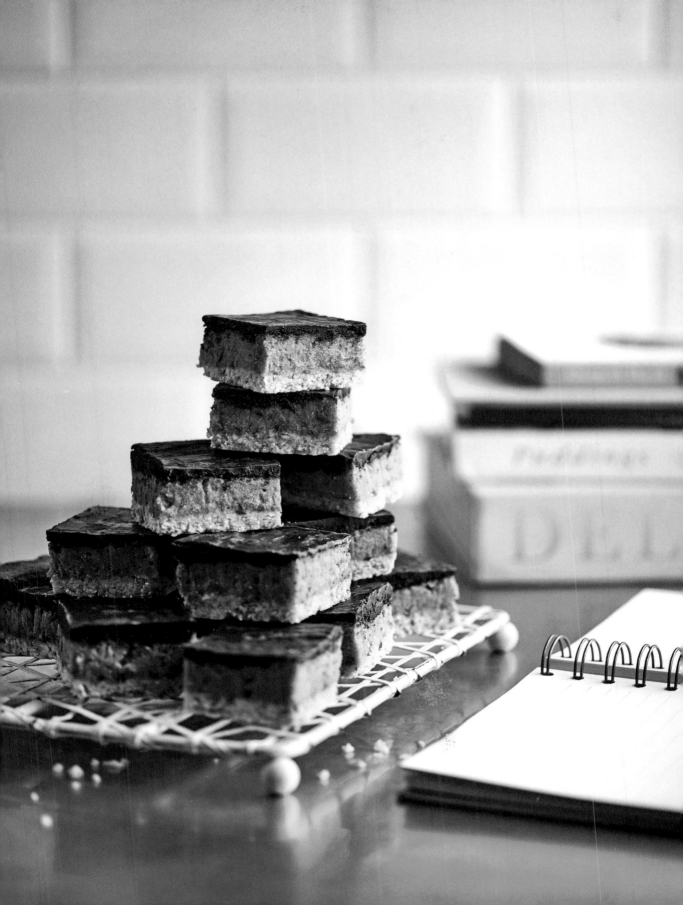

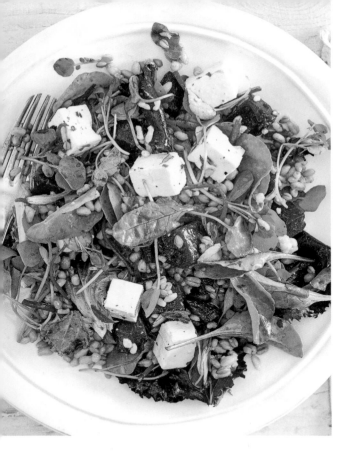
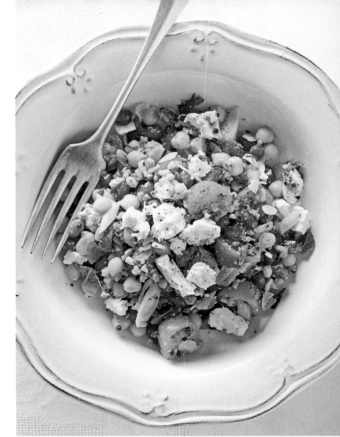
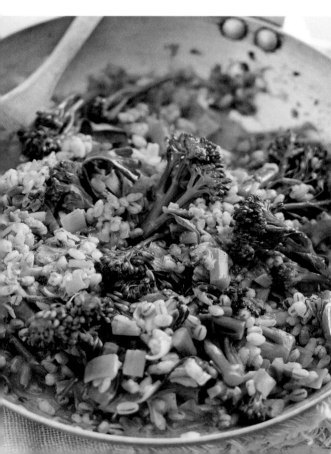
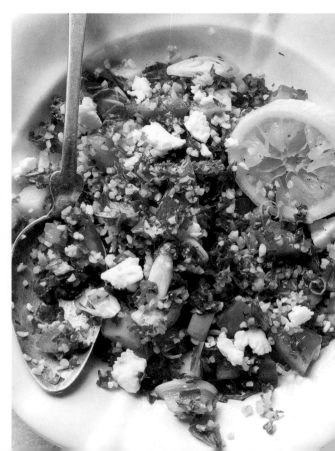

Chapter 3:

GORGEOUS GRAINS

· ·

A healthy, well-running digestive system is key to good health – helping to keep skin clear and your body in good working order. To achieve this fibre is an essential component of a superfood diet and that's why our recipes include whole-grains rather than the refined, processed white varieties, which disrupt blood sugar and are stripped of their superfood goodness.

There are two main types of fibre – soluble and insoluble. The oats and barley in our Three-grain porridge (page 78) carry a true superfood punch because they're an excellent source of a special type called beta-glucan. This soluble form is gentler on the digestive system and helps manage cholesterol levels.

Including more whole-grains doesn't mean lots of bulky dishes. We've used brown rice in our Chunky vegetable & brown rice soup (page 94). Brown rice is rich in the mineral manganese, which helps produce energy from the protein and carbs you eat. We've also included quinoa – known as a pseudo-grain, quinoa is actually a seed. It creates a lighter dish than say couscous or pasta yet is still a good source of fibre as well as B vitamins and minerals including zinc.

As a general guide keep the carb portion on your plate to about a fist size of nutritious whole-grains.

Help-yourself grain fridge salad

This salad will sit happily in the fridge for two to three days, ready for on-the-go lunches or quick dinners.

PREP 25 mins NO COOK 4

- finely grated zest and juice 2 lemons
- 3 tbsp extra virgin olive oil
- 1 tbsp clear honey
- 2 tbsp tahini
- 250g pouch of cooked wholegrains
- 400 g can chickpeas, drained
- 1 pomegranate, seeds removed
- 200g cherry tomatoes (a mix of red and yellow looks attractive), halved
- large bunch mint or parsley (or a mixture), leaves picked and roughly chopped
- 50g toasted flaked almonds
- bunch spring onions, finely sliced on an angle
- 200g pack feta, crumbled

1 In a large bowl or sealable container, whisk the lemon zest and juice, oil, honey, tahini and some seasoning. Squeeze the grain pouch to separate the grains, then tip into the bowl along with the chickpeas, pomegranate seeds, tomatoes, herbs, almonds, spring onions and half the feta.

2 Toss everything together in the bowl to coat in the dressing, then crumble over the remaining feta. Serve in bowls straight away, or cover the container and put in the fridge. Eat within 3 days.

Nutrition: *per serving*
kcal 580 fat 36g saturates 10g carbs 35g sugars 11g fibre 7g protein 24g salt 2.6g

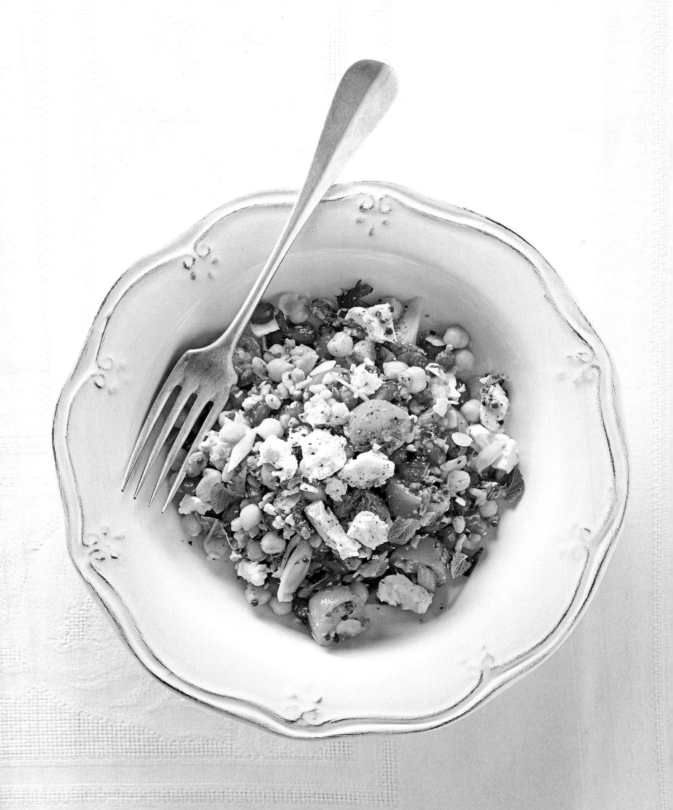

Three-grain porridge mix

Make up a batch of this porridge mix, ready for healthy breakfasts in a flash.

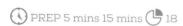 PREP 5 mins 15 mins 18

- 300g oatmeal
- 300g spelt flakes
- 300g barley flakes
- agave nectar and sliced strawberries, to serve (optional)

1 Working in batches, toast the oatmeal, spelt flakes and barley in a large, dry frying pan for 5 mins until golden, then leave to cool and store in an airtight container.

2 When you want to eat it, simply combine 50g of the porridge mixture in a saucepan with 300ml milk or water. Cook for 5 mins, stirring occasionally, then top with a drizzle of honey and strawberries, if you like (optional). Will keep for 6 months.

Nutrition: *per serving*
kcal 179 fat 2g saturates 0g carbs 32g sugars 1g fibre 4g protein 7g salt 0g

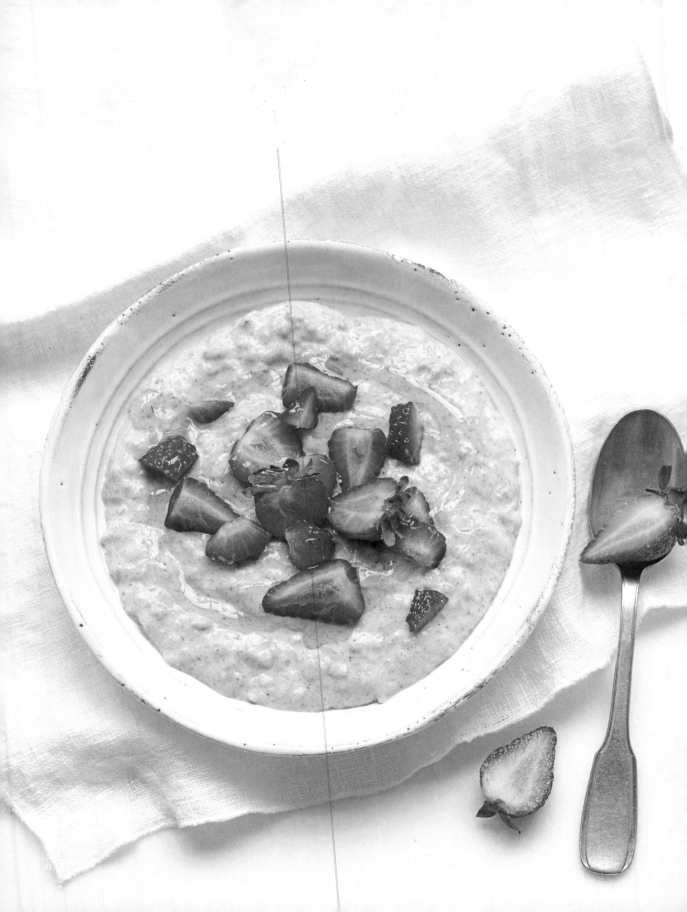

Cardamom & peach quinoa porridge

This porridge will keep you going until lunchtime, serve with whatever fruit is in season.

PREP 3 mins COOK 20 mins 2

- 75g quinoa
- 25g porridge oats
- 4 cardamom pods
- 250ml unsweetened almond milk
- 2 ripe peaches, cut into slices
- 1 tsp maple syrup

1 Put the quinoa, oats and cardamom pods in a small saucepan with 250ml water and 100ml of the almond milk. Bring to the boil, then simmer gently for 15 mins, stirring occasionally.

2 Pour in the remaining almond milk and cook for 5 mins more until creamy.

3 Remove the cardamom pods, spoon into bowls or jars, and top with the peaches and maple syrup.

Nutrition: *per serving*
kcal 231 fat 4g saturates 1g carbs 37g sugars 10g fibre 6g protein 8g salt 0.2g

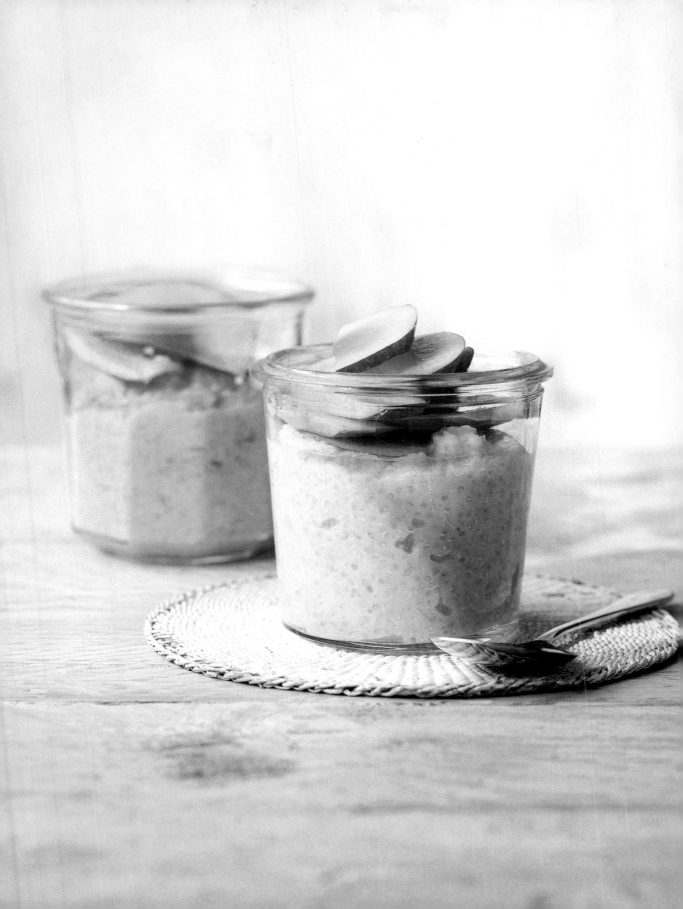

Breakfast muffins

Make up a batch of the healthy muffins and store in a cake tin for up to 3 days. They also freeze well – wrap individually in cling film and bring out of the freezer the night before you want to eat them.

PREP 15 mins COOK 30 mins 4

- 2 large eggs
- 150ml pot natural yogurt
- 50ml rapeseed oil
- 100g apple sauce or puréed apples (find with the baby food)
- 1 ripe banana, mashed
- 4 tbsp clear honey
- 1 tsp vanilla extract
- 200g wholemeal or mixed wholegrain flour
- 50g rolled oats, plus extra for sprinkling
- 1½ tsp baking powder
- 1½ tsp bicarbonate of soda
- 1½ tsp cinnamon
- 100g blueberries
- 2 tbsp mixed seeds (we used pumpkin, sunflower and flaxseed)

1 Heat oven to 180C/160C fan/gas 4. Line a 12-hole muffin tin with 12 large muffin cases. In a jug, mix the eggs, yogurt, oil, apple sauce, banana, honey and vanilla. Tip the remaining ingredients, except the seeds, into a large bowl, add a pinch of salt and mix to combine.

2 Pour the wet ingredients into the dry and mix briefly until you have a smooth batter – don't overmix as this will make the muffins heavy. Divide the batter among the cases. Sprinkle the muffins with the extra oats and the seeds. Bake for 25–30 mins until golden and well risen, and a skewer inserted into the centre of a muffin comes out clean. Remove from the oven, transfer to a wire rack and leave to cool. Can be stored in a sealed container for up to 3 days.

Nutrition: *per muffin*
kcal 188 fat 7g saturates 1g carbs 24g sugars 10g fibre 3g protein 5g salt 0.6g

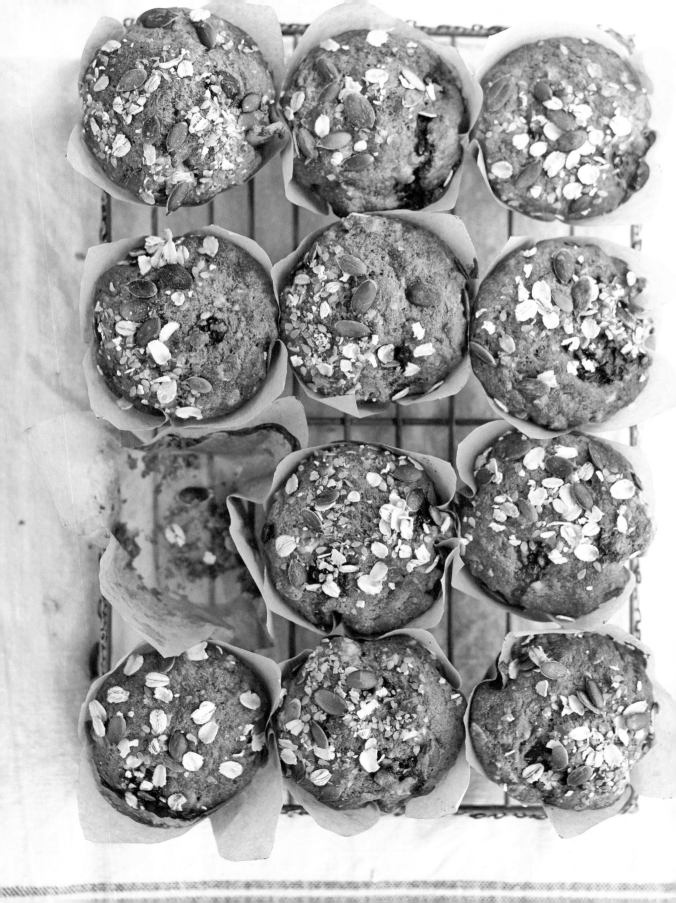

Tuna, avocado & quinoa salad

Quinoa is actually a seed, but can be used as you would a grain in salads. It's high in protein, fibre and magnesium.

PREP 5 mins COOK 25 mins 2

- 100g quinoa
- 3 tbsp extra virgin olive oil
- juice 1 lemon
- ½ tbsp white wine vinegar
- 120g can tuna, drained
- 1 avocado, stoned, peeled and cut into chunks
- 200g cherry tomatoes on the vine, halved
- 50g feta, crumbled
- 50g baby spinach
- 2 tbsp mixed seeds, toasted

1 Rinse the quinoa under cold water. Tip into a saucepan, cover with water and bring to the boil. Reduce the heat and simmer for 15 mins until the grains have swollen but still have some bite. Drain, then transfer to a bowl to cool slightly.
2 Meanwhile, in a jug, combine the oil, lemon juice and vinegar with some seasoning.
3 Once the quinoa has cooled, mix with the dressing and all the remaining ingredients and season. Divide between plates or lunchboxes.

Nutrition: *per serving*
kcal 663 fat 44g saturates 10g carbs 34g sugars 7g fibre 8g protein 28g salt 1.1g

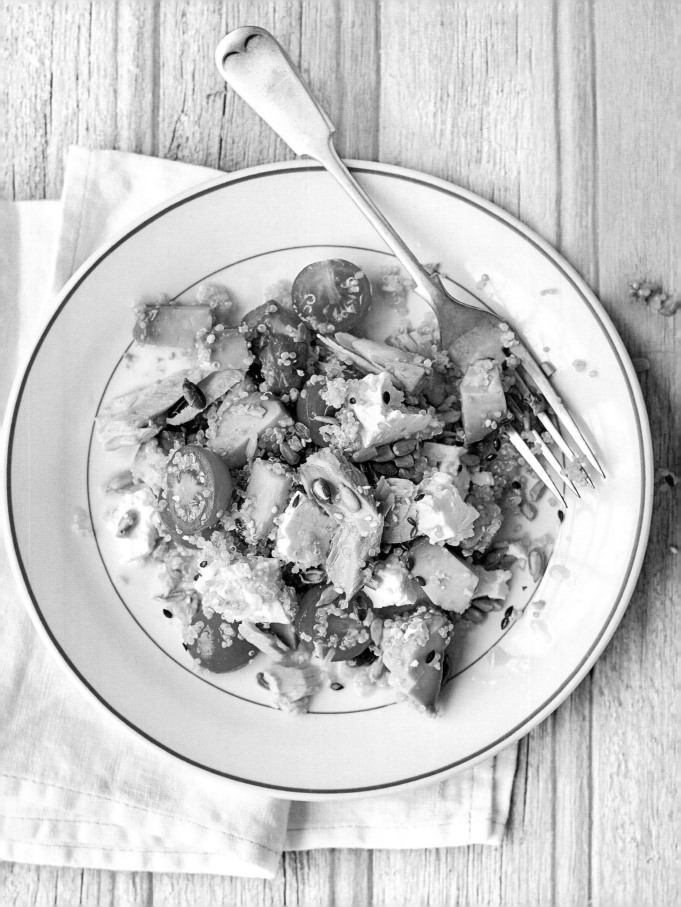

Barley & broccoli risotto with lemon & basil

Look out for wholegrain pearl barley for this recipe, as regular pearl barley has had many of the nutrients stripped away. It makes a great alternative to risotto rice, with a nice nutty texture.

PREP 10 mins COOK 35 mins plus soaking 2

- 100g wholegrain pearl barley
- 2 tsp reduced-salt vegetable bouillon powder
- 2 tbsp rapeseed oil
- 1 large leek, chopped
- 2 garlic cloves
- small pack basil
- generous squeeze of lemon juice
- 125g Tenderstem broccoli

1 Pour a litre of cold water over the barley, cover and leave to soak overnight.
2 The next day, drain the barley, reserve the liquid and use it to make 500ml vegetable bouillon. Heat half the oil in a non-stick pan, add the leek and cook briefly to soften. Tip half into a bowl, then add the barley and bouillon to the pan, cover and simmer for 20 mins.
3 Meanwhile, add the garlic, basil, remaining oil, the lemon juice and 3 tbsp water to the leeks in the bowl, and blitz to a paste with a stick blender
4 When the barley has cooked for 20 mins, add the broccoli to the pan and cook for 5–10 mins more until both are tender. Stir in the basil purée, heat very briefly (to retain the fragrance), then spoon into bowls to serve.

Nutrition: *per serving*
kcal 378 fat 14g saturates 1g carbs 49g sugars 5g fibre 7g protein 11g salt 0.1g

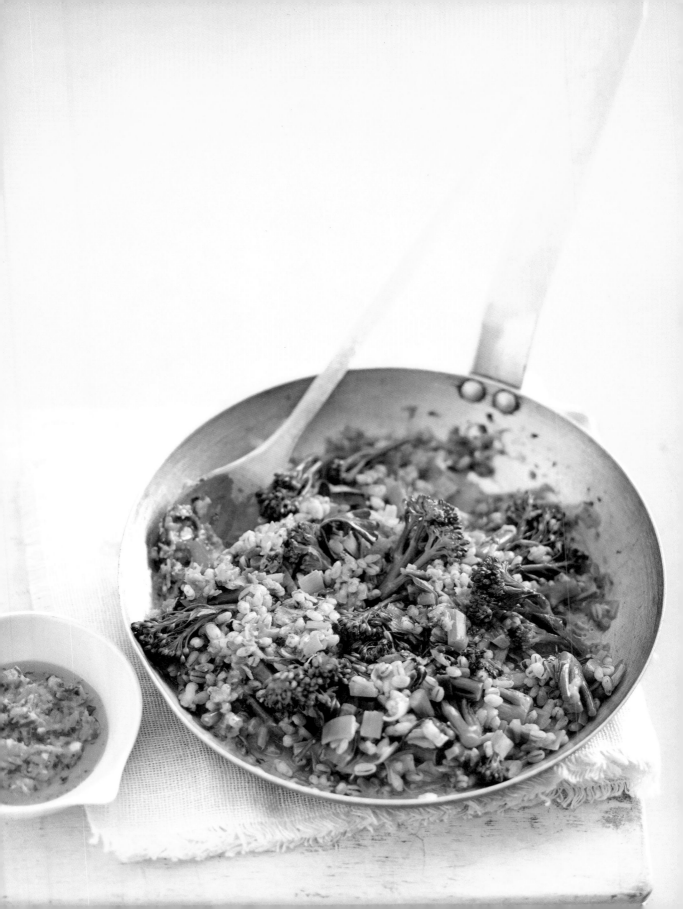

Beetroot, feta & grain salad

This recipe barely even needs instructions, but sometimes it's good to have a grab and go standby recipe up your sleeve. Add some toasted seeds for extra crunch and protein, if you like.

PREP 2 mins NO COOK 2

- 110g bag mixed salad leaves
- 100g marinated feta in olive oil
- 250g cooked beetroot, chopped
- 1 ready-to-eat mixed wholegrain pouch

1 Put all the ingredients in a large bowl and toss together with some seasoning, The oil in the feta will create a dressing for the salad.

Nutrition: *per serving*
kcal 509 fat 21g saturates 8g carbs 59g sugars 24g fibre 10g protein 17g salt 2.3g

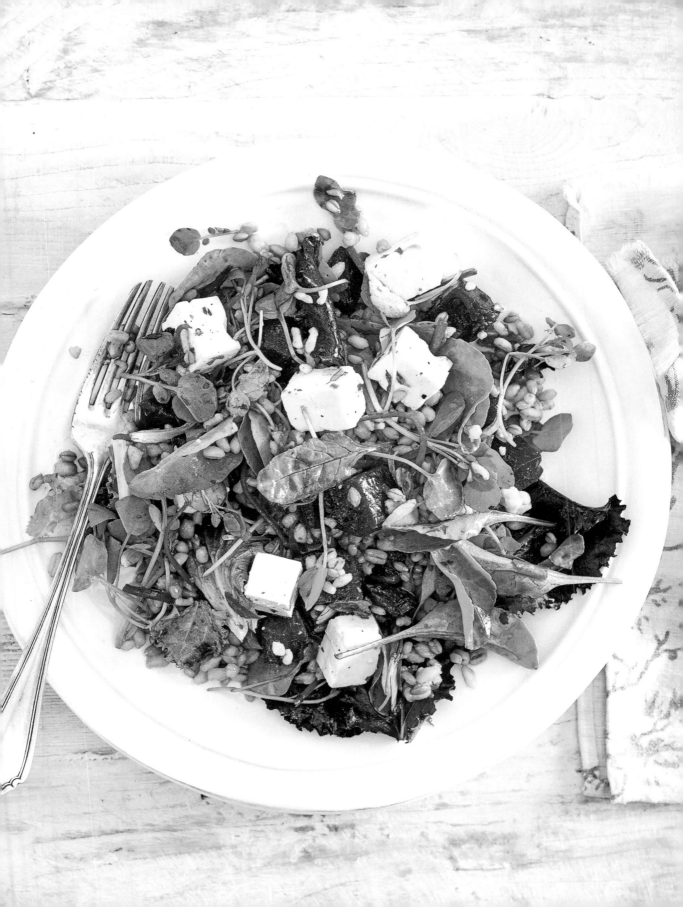

Bulghar wheat, date & clementine salad

Use bulghar wheat in place of couscous where you can, it is a whole-grain and therefore much higher in beneficial nutrients such as protein and fibre.

PREP 15 mins COOK 10 mins 2

- 140g bulghar wheat
- 1 tsp ground allspice
- 1 tsp ground cumin
- 6 stoned dates, chopped
- small handful parsley, chopped
- 400g can chickpeas, drained
- 2 tbsp flaked toasted almonds
- 100g bag baby spinach
- 2 clementines, peel removed, sliced

FOR THE DRESSING
- juice 1 lemon
- 2 tbsp sherry vinegar
- 2 tbsp extra virgin olive oil

1 Put the bulghar wheat and spices in a large bowl, season with salt and pour over 140ml boiling water. Cover with cling film and leave to sit for 10 mins. Fluff with a fork, then add the chopped dates, parsley, chickpeas and most of the almonds. Pour the dressing ingredients into a glass jar with a fitted lid and add some seasoning. Shake well and pour over the salad.

2 Just before eating, mix the spinach through, top with the clementine slices and scatter with the remaining almonds.

Nutrition: *per serving*
kcal 765 fat 23g saturates 3g carbs 114g sugars 42g fibre 10g protein 19g salt 1.1g

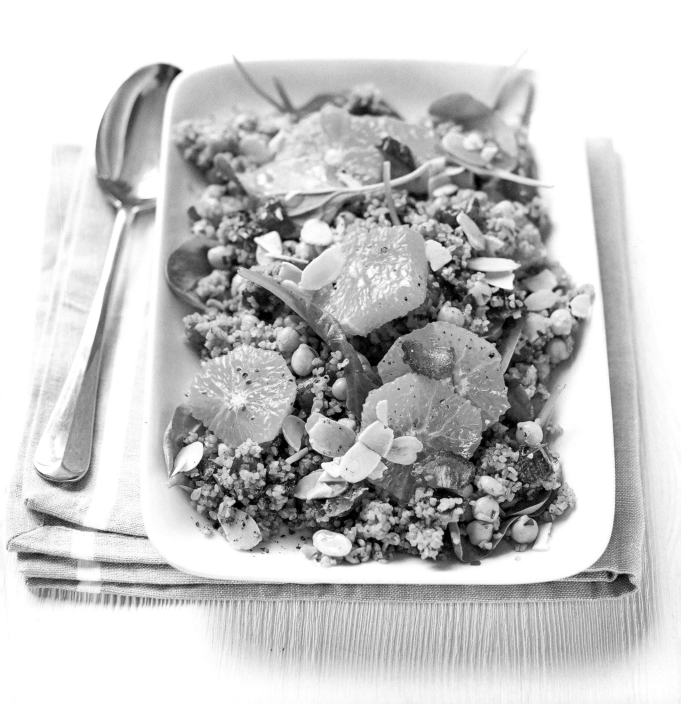

Kale tabbouleh

Tabblouleh is a chopped herb and grain salad. This recipe also contains kale, boosting its superfood credentials.

PREP 15 mins COOK 15 mins 6

- 100g bulghar wheat
- 100g kale
- large bunch mint, roughly chopped
- bunch spring onions, sliced
- ½ cucumber, diced
- 4 tomatoes, deseeded and chopped
- pinch of ground cinnamon
- pinch of ground allspice
- 6 tbsp olive oil
- juice and zest ½ lemon
- 100g feta cheese, crumbled
- 4 Baby Gem lettuce leaves, separated, to serve

1 Tip the bulghar wheat into a heatproof bowl and just cover with boiling water, then cover with cling film and set aside for 10–15 mins or until tender. Put the kale in a food processor and pulse to finely chop.

2 Stir the kale, mint, spring onions, cucumber and tomatoes through the bulghar wheat. Season with the cinnamon and allspice, then dress with the olive oil and lemon juice to taste. Scatter over the lemon zest and feta. To serve, let everyone scoop the salad onto leaves of Baby Gem lettuce.

Nutrition: *per serving*
kcal 235 fat 15g saturates 4g carbs 17g sugars 4g fibre 2g protein 6g salt 0.7g

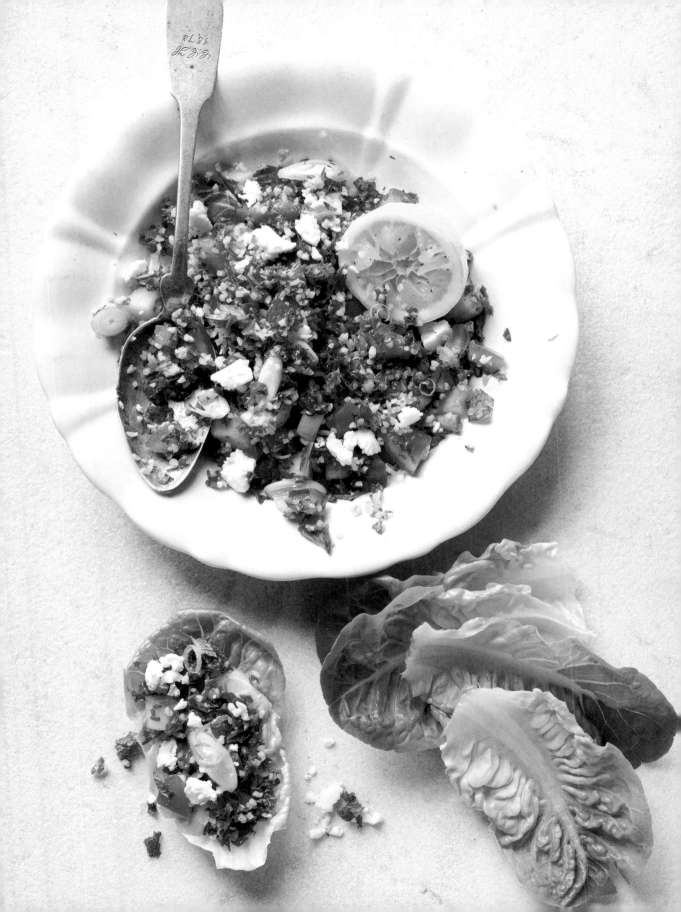

Chunky vegetable & brown rice soup

Double the quantity of this soup and stash a few portions in the freezer for a rainy day.

PREP 18 mins COOK 50 mins 4

- 2 tbsp extra virgin rapeseed oil
- 1 medium onion, halved and sliced
- 2 garlic cloves, finely sliced
- 2 celery sticks, trimmed and thinly sliced
- 2 medium carrots, cut into chunks
- 2 medium parsnips, cut into chunks
- 1 tbsp finely chopped thyme leaves
- 100g wholegrain rice
- 2 medium leeks, sliced
- ½ small pack parsley, to garnish

1 Heat the oil in a large non-stick pan and add the onion, garlic, celery, carrots, parsnips and thyme. Cover with a lid and cook gently for 15 mins, stirring occasionally, until the onions are softened and beginning to colour. Add the rice and pour in 1.2 litres cold water or stock. Bring to the boil, then reduce the heat to a simmer and cook, uncovered, for 15 mins, stirring occasionally.

2 Season the soup with plenty of ground black pepper and salt to taste, then stir in the leeks. Return to a gentle simmer and cook for a further 5 mins or until the leeks have softened. Adjust the seasoning to taste and blitz half the soup with a stick blender, leaving the other half chunky, if you like. Top with the parsley and serve in deep bowls.

Nutrition: *per serving*
kcal 261 fat 8g saturates 1g carbs 37g sugars 11g fibre 10g protein 5g salt 0.5g

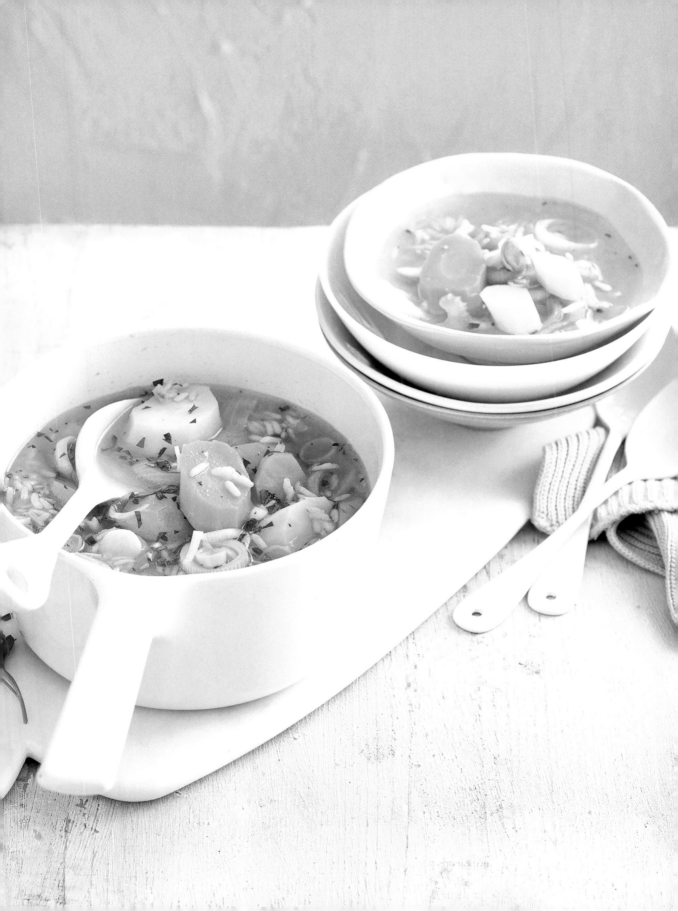

Black bean, tofu, avocado & rice bowl

Cooked rice and grain pouches can provide you with a speedy dinner solution if you're short for time.

PREP 20 mins COOK 25 mins 4

- 2 tbsp olive or extra virgin rapeseed oil
- 1 red onion, chopped
- 3 garlic cloves, crushed
- 2 tsp ground cumin
- 2 x 400g cans black beans, drained and rinsed
- zest 2 limes, then 1 juiced, the other cut into wedges to serve
- 396g pack tofu, halved through the centre, then chopped into small chunks
- 2 tsp smoked paprika
- 2 x 200g pouches cooked brown rice
- 2 small ripe avocados, halved, stoned, peeled and chopped
- small bunch coriander, leaves only
- 1 red chilli, thinly sliced (optional)

1 Heat the grill to High. Heat 1 tbsp oil in a frying pan, add the onion and cook, stirring, for 5 mins or so until soft. Add the garlic and sizzle for 30 secs more, then stir in the cumin and black beans. Cook for 5 mins until the beans start to pop and are hot through. Stir through the lime zest and juice, and season.

2 While the beans cook, put the tofu in a bowl and gently toss through the remaining oil, the paprika and some seasoning. Line a baking tray with foil and arrange the tofu on top. Cook under the grill for 5 mins each side until charred all over.

3 Heat the rice following pack instructions, then divide among bowls. Top with the beans, tofu, avocado, coriander and a wedge of lime. Add a few slices of chilli too, if you like it spicy.

Nutrition: *per serving*
kcal 546 fat 25g saturates 4g carbs 48g sugars 4g fibre 14g protein 25g salt 0.8g

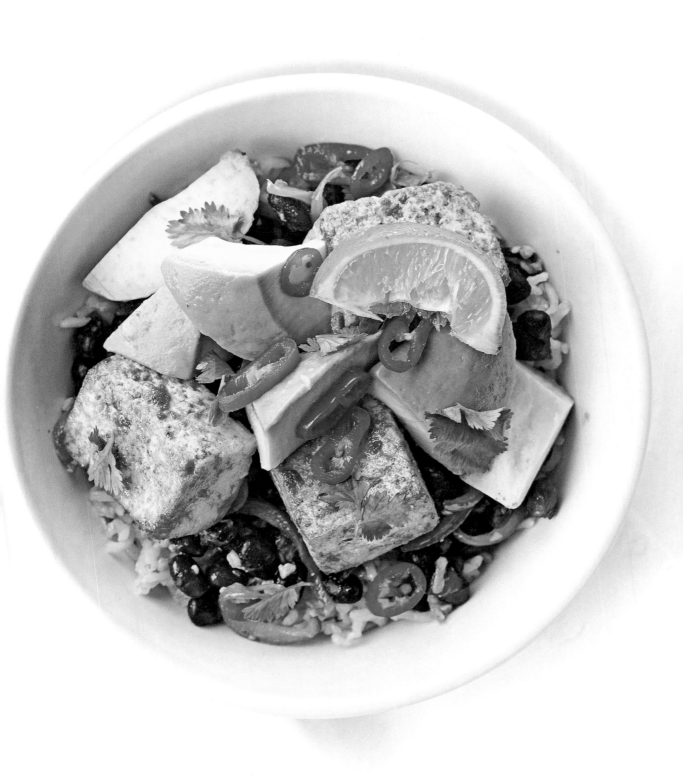

Herby rice with roasted veg, chickpeas & halloumi

This vegetarian dinner is high in protein, whole-grains and colourful veg. The halloumi makes a nice alternative to meat.

PREP 15 mins COOK 35 mins 4

- 2 red onions, cut into chunky wedges
- 3 peppers, sliced (we used green, red and yellow)
- 3 courgettes (about 600g), cut into batons
- 5 tbsp olive oil
- 200g brown basmati rice
- small pack flat-leaf parsley
- 85g cashew nuts
- 1 garlic clove, crushed
- 400g can chickpeas, drained and rinsed
- 200g halloumi, cut into chunky cubes

1 Heat oven to 200C/180C fan/gas 6. Put the red onions, peppers and courgettes in a large roasting tin, toss in 2 tbsp oil and season. (You may need to do this in 2 tins.) Pop in the oven and cook for 25 mins until the veg is tender and beginning to turn golden.

2 Meanwhile, cook the rice following pack instructions. Whizz together the parsley, cashew nuts, remaining oil, the garlic and seasoning to make a pesto. Stir the chickpeas and halloumi into the roasted veg and cook for 10 mins more. Fork the parsley pesto through the rice, spoon over the veg and serve.

Nutrition: *per serving*
kcal 782 fat 40g saturates 13g carbs 70g sugars 17g fibre 1g protein 29g salt 1.9g

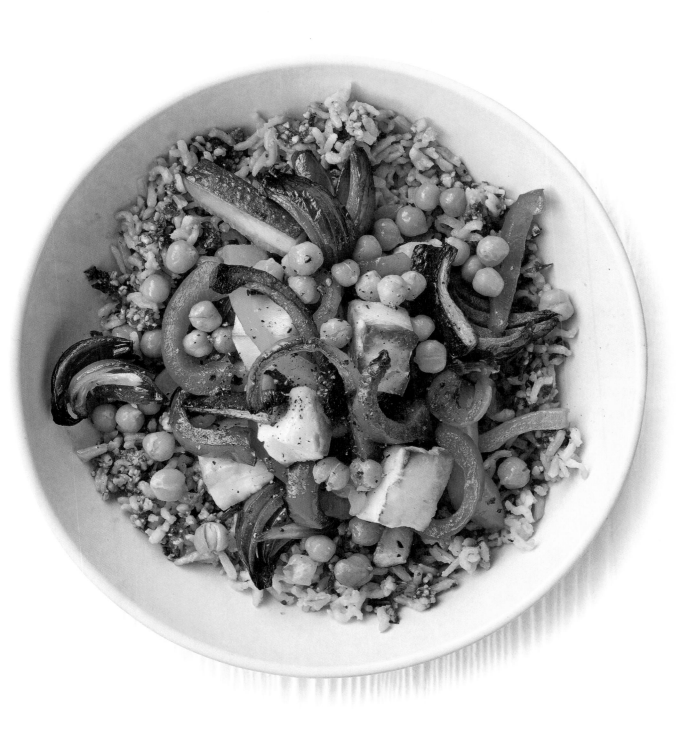

One-pan tikka salmon with jewelled rice

Marinate salmon with yogurt and curry paste, then cook with brown rice in one pan to steam the fish until tender and flaky.

PREP 10 mins COOK 1 hour 3

- 3 tbsp tikka curry paste
- 150ml pot natural yogurt
- 3 salmon fillets, skinned
- 2 tsp olive oil
- 1 large red onion, chopped
- 1 tsp turmeric
- 50g soft dried apricots, chopped
- 200g brown basmati rice
- 100g pack pomegranate seeds
- small pack coriander, leaves picked

1 Combine 1 tbsp of the curry paste with 2 tbsp yogurt. Season the salmon and smear the yogurt paste all over the fillets, then set aside. Heat the oil in a large pan (with a lid) and add the onion. Boil the kettle. Cook the onion for 5 mins to soften, and stir in the remaining curry paste then cook for 1 min more. Add the turmeric, apricots and rice, season well and give everything a good stir. Pour in 800ml water from the kettle. Bring to a boil, and simmer for 15 mins. Cover with a lid, lower the heat to a gentle simmer and cook for 15 mins more.

2 Uncover the rice and give it a good stir. Put the salmon fillets on top of the rice and re-cover the pan. Turn the heat to its lowest setting and leave undisturbed for 15–20 mins more until the salmon and rice are perfectly cooked. Scatter over the pomegranate seeds and coriander, and serve with the yogurt.

Nutrition: *per serving*
kcal 688 fat 25g saturates 4g carbs 69g sugars 22g fibre 8g protein 45g salt 0.9g

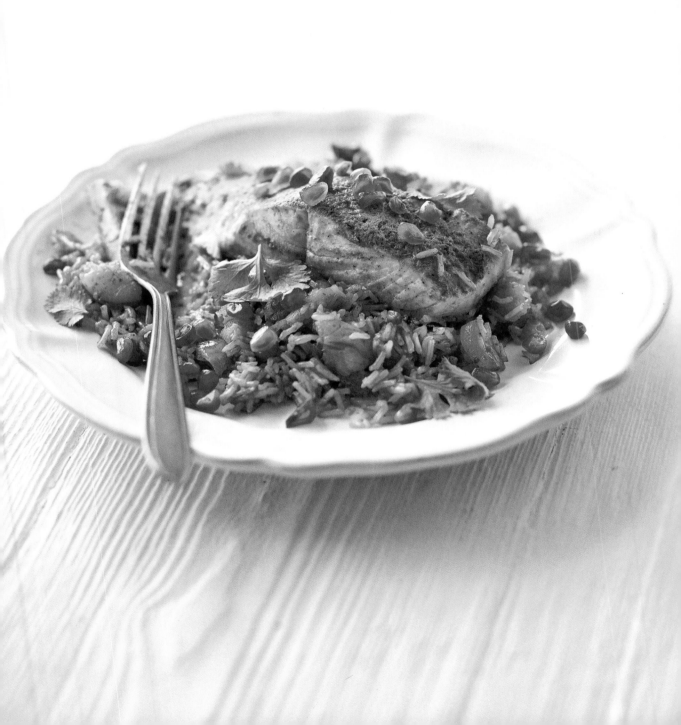

Turkey pilaf with saffron & goji berries

This is the ultimate recipe for brain health, packed with brain-boosting nutrients like cinnamon, almonds and goji berries.

PREP 15 mins COOK 40 mins 2

- generous pinch of saffron
- 3 tsp extra virgin rapeseed oil
- 200g diced skinless turkey thigh
- 85g brown basmati rice
- ½ tsp ground cinnamon
- 1 tsp vegetable bouillon
- 3 celery sticks, finely chopped
- 1 tbsp thyme leaves
- 1 tbsp dried goji berries
- 1 medium onion, halved and very thinly sliced
- 2 large garlic cloves, chopped
- 100g baby spinach leaves
- 25g flaked almonds

1 Pour 2 tbsp boiling water over the saffron and set aside to infuse. Heat 2 tsp of the oil in a large, non-stick sauté pan with a lid, then add the turkey and fry for 5 mins, stirring frequently, until it starts to brown.

2 Stir the rice and cinnamon into the pan, then pour in 400ml boiling water and the bouillon, and stir well. Add the celery, thyme, goji berries and lots of ground black pepper. Cover the pan tightly to prevent steam escaping, and cook over a low heat for 20 mins.

3 Meanwhile, heat the remaining oil in a non-stick pan and add the onion. When it starts to soften, cover the pan for 5 mins to steam it a little more. Take off the lid and slowly fry for 12–15 mins until golden, stirring frequently.

4 After the rice has cooked for 20 mins, check the water level – if the rice is still too nutty and the liquid has all been absorbed, add up to 100ml more water. Stir in the saffron, cover again, and cook for 5–10 mins until the rice is tender.

5 Add the garlic and spinach, cook briefly to wilt the leaves, then turn off the heat. Toss through the fried onions and almonds. Cover the pan and leave to rest for 5 mins before serving.

Nutrition: *per serving*
kcal 454 fat 16g saturates 2g carbs 42g sugars 10g fibre 7g protein 32g salt 0.6g

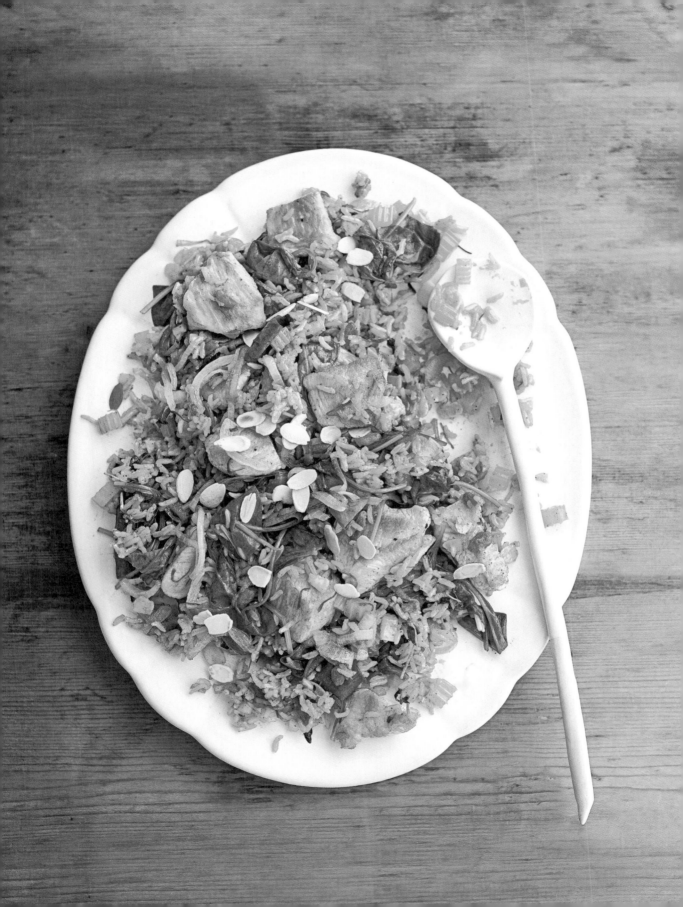

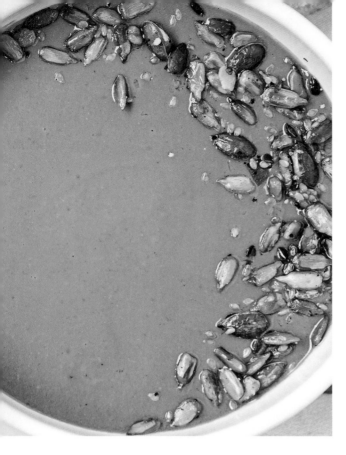
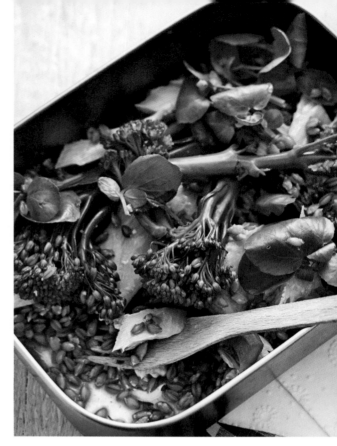
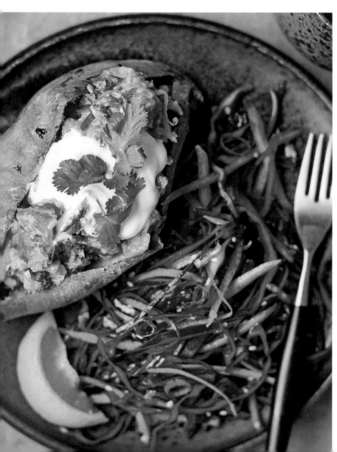
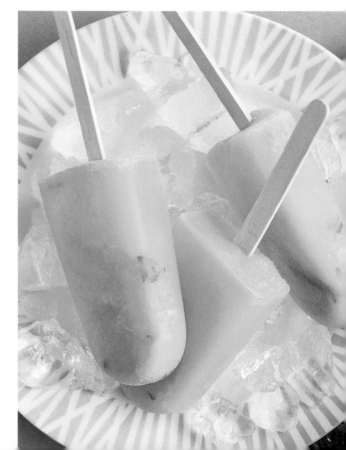

Chapter 4:

RAINBOW FRUIT & VEG

The foundation of any superfood diet has to be a varied and wide selection of fruit and veg. All the wonderful colours represent the different antioxidants and phyto-chemicals that fruit and veg contain, including anthocyanins, polyphenols, flavonoids and carotenoids. These compounds protect against modern day diseases, but each in a slightly different way. That's why we're encouraging you to eat the rainbow. Enjoying a wide selection of fruit and veg can benefit health from better moods to a strengthened immunity.

Almost all red fruit and veg contain the carotenoid, lycopene, which minimizes the damage caused by UV light on the skin. While leafy greens like watercress, kale and spinach are rich in lutein, which is important for healthy vision, and zeaxanthin, which may reduce the risk of certain cancers. The deep colour of blueberries is due to anthocyanins, which boost memory, maintain firm skin and help preserve flexible, healthy arteries. When out of season choose red cabbage, which contains the same valuable compounds.

We've included a number of beetroot recipes in our collection – this root veg is effective at lowering blood pressure and helps repair muscles after exercise. Being rich in nitrates, beetroot improves blood oxygenation, so a portion of beetroot or a glass of its juice will help you go that extra mile.

Super-green fish cakes

This is a great healthy recipe to feed to kids. Serve with extra peas and lemon wedges for squeezing over.

PREP 30 mins COOK 30 mins plus chilling 4

- 2 medium potatoes, peeled and chopped
- 1 medium sweet potato, peeled and chopped
- 1 small head of broccoli, cut into florets
- 100g frozen peas, plus extra, cooked, to serve
- small bunch parsley, roughly chopped
- zest 1 lemon, plus wedges to serve
- 2 tsp Dijon mustard
- 225g pack (about 3 fillets) smoked mackerel, flaked
- 5 tbsp plain flour, plus a little for dusting
- 3 tbsp vegetable, sunflower or extra virgin rapeseed oil, for frying

1 Put the potatoes and sweet potatoes in a large pan of cold, salted water, cover and bring to the boil. Simmer for 10 mins until starting to soften around the edges but not completely tender. Add the broccoli and cook for 4 mins more, then add the peas and cook for another 30 secs. Drain and leave everything in the colander to drain and cool completely. Can be kept in the fridge overnight.

2 Tip the veg and potatoes into a food processor. Add the parsley, lemon zest, mustard, mackerel, flour and some seasoning. Blend until the mixture is finely chopped and starts to clump together. Remove the blade from the mixer and shape into 8 cakes, dusting your hands and the cakes in flour. Put the cakes on a plate and chill for 30 mins or until they have firmed up, Can be wrapped and frozen for up to 2 months.

3 Heat the oil in a large non-stick frying pan. Cook the cakes for 5–8 mins each side until golden, crispy and hot throughout. Serve with extra peas and lemon wedges.

Nutrition: *per serving*
kcal 492 fat 24g saturates 4g carbs 43g sugars 8g fibre 9g protein 20g salt 1.5g

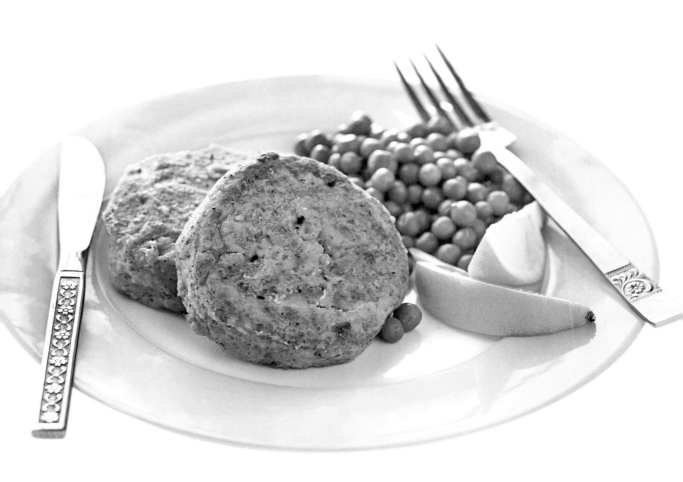

Trout & spelt salad with watercress

If you want to save time, use a ready cooked pouch of spelt for this easy salad.

⏱ PREP 5 mins COOK 5 mins 🍽 1

- 85g thin-stemmed broccoli
- juice ½ orange
- 1 tbsp chopped flat leaf parsley
- 140g cooked spelt
- 140g hot-smoked trout, flaked
- large handful watercress

Steam or boil the broccoli for 3 mins until al dente. Mix together the orange juice, parsley and spelt, then top with the broccoli, trout and watercress.

Nutrition: *per serving*
kcal 415 fat 10g saturates 2g carbs 36g sugars 3g fibre 10g protein 41g salt 2.6g

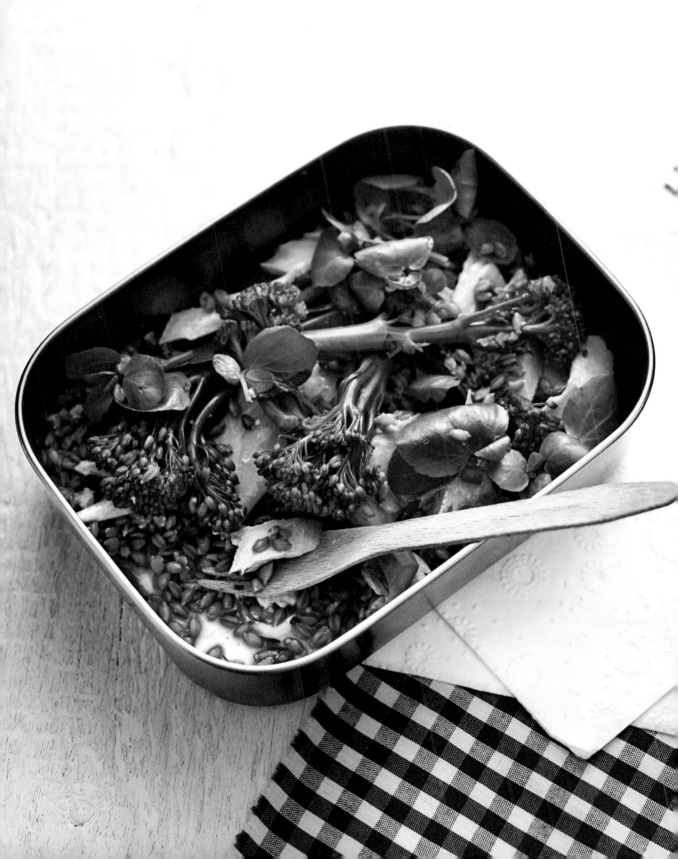

Spinach & watercress soup

This is a great soup to make for a quick lunch, the ingredients are only briefly cooked so the greens retain most of their nutrients and their bright green colour.

PREP 5 mins COOK 5 mins 1

- 100g spinach
- 100g watercress
- 1 spring onion, sliced
- 100ml vegetable stock
- ½ avocado, stoned and peeled
- 100g cooked wholegrain rice
- juice ½ lemon
- 2 tbsp mixed seeds, plus extra to serve

Put the spinach, watercress, spring onion, vegetable stock, avocado, cooked rice, lemon juice and mixed seeds in a blender with some seasoning. Whizz until smooth. Heat until piping hot. Scatter over some toasted seeds if you want added crunch.

Nutrition: *per serving*
kcal 457 fat 26g saturates 6g carbs 33g sugars 2g fibre 9g protein 18g salt 0.5g

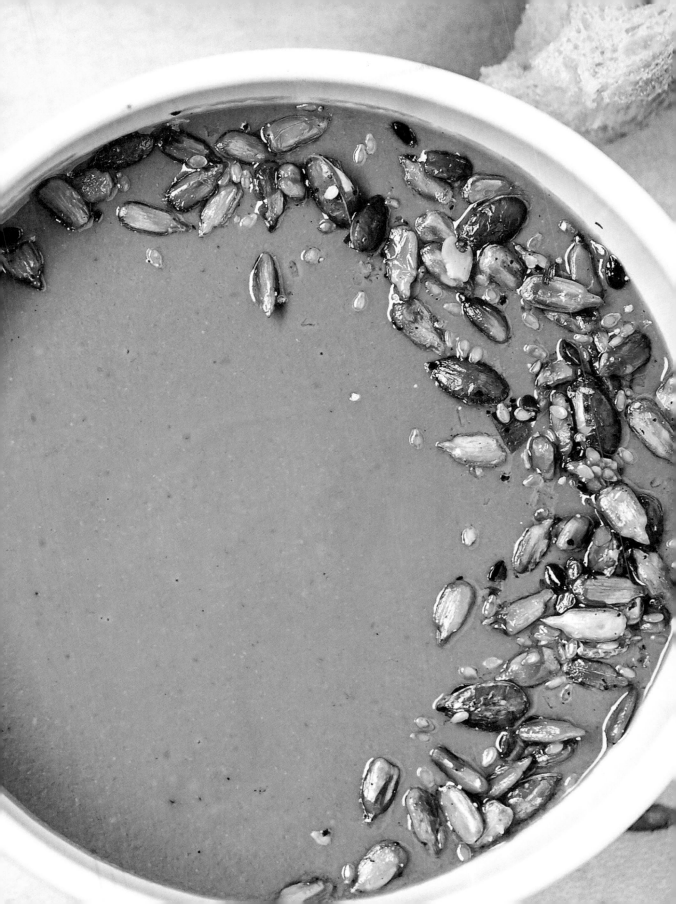

Watermelon & spinach super salad

This fresh salad makes a wonderful lunch on its own, or would make a nice side dish to serve with roast lamb.

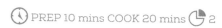 PREP 10 mins COOK 20 mins 2

- 100g quinoa
- 2 tbsp pumpkin seeds
- ½ small watermelon, skin and seeds removed, cut into chunks
- 80g baby spinach
- 1 ripe avocado, peeled and sliced
- ½ small pack mint, finely chopped
- 50g feta, crumbled
- juice 1 lime
- 1 punnet salad cress

1 Rinse the quinoa, then put it in a pan with a fitted lid and cover with 200ml water. Cook, covered, over a medium heat for 15 mins or until fluffy and the water has been absorbed. Fork through to separate the grains, then leave to cool.

2 Meanwhile, heat a frying pan over a medium heat and toast the pumpkin seeds for 1 min or until they start to pop. Tip into a serving bowl or on a platter with the watermelon, spinach, avocado, mint and feta. Toss through the quinoa, then squeeze over the lime juice with a pinch of seasoning. Top with the cress and serve.

Nutrition: *per serving*
kcal 507 fat 25g saturates 7g carbs 48g sugars 18g fibre 8g protein 19g salt 0.8g

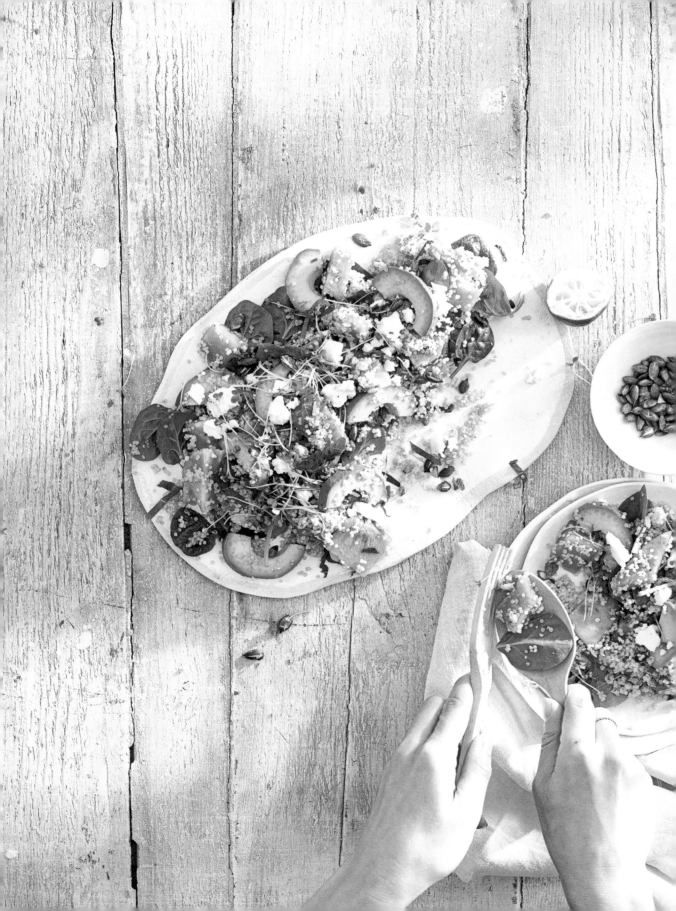

Pods & sods with watercress

An easy way to serve greens with your Sunday roast.

PREP 5 mins COOK 5 mins 6

- bunch of asparagus, woody ends removed, each spear sliced into 3 pieces on an angle
- 100g fresh or frozen podded broad beans, skins removed
- 100g fresh or frozen peas
- 100g frozen soya or edamame beans
- 3 spring onions, each sliced into 3 pieces on an angle
- ½ small pack mint, leaves torn
- 100g bag watercress

FOR THE DRESSING
- 1 tsp Dijon mustard
- 4 tbsp olive oil
- 1 tsp white wine vinegar

1 Bring a large pan of salted water to the boil. Drop in the asparagus, bring back to the boil, then add all the beans, the peas and spring onions. Bring to the boil again, then drain and cool quickly by running under cold water.
2 To make the dressing, mix the mustard with the oil, vinegar and some seasoning. On a large platter, mix all the vegetables with the mint, watercress and a splash of dressing.

Nutrition: *per serving*
kcal 137 fat 9g saturates 1g carbs 6g sugars 2g fibre 5g protein 6g salt 0.1g

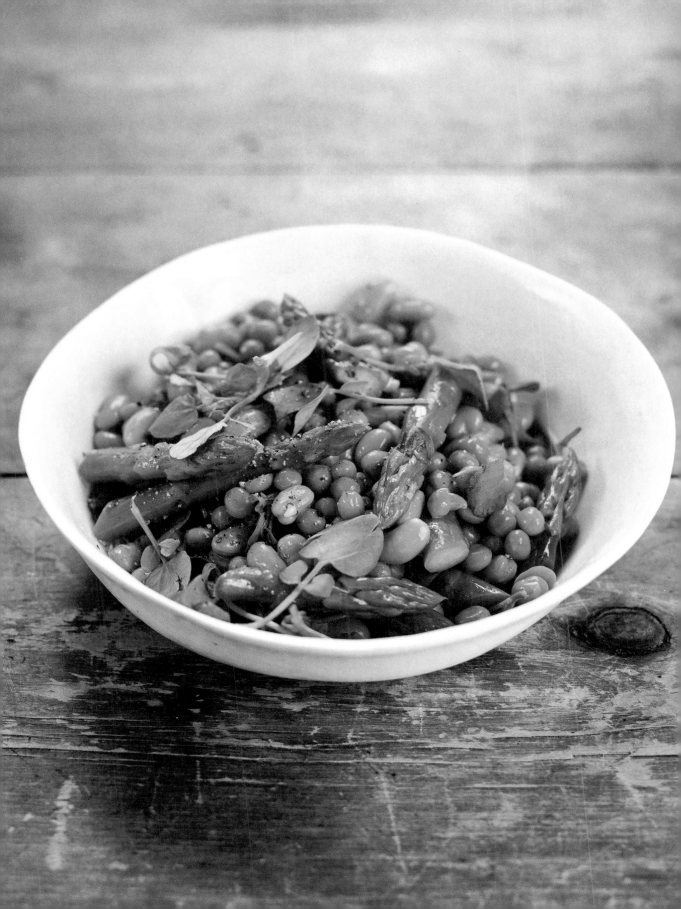

Nutty watercress pesto

Toss this nutrient packed pesto through cooked tagliatelle, or try courgetti if you want to up your intake of greens.

PREP 15 mins NO COOK 4

- 100g pack watercress
- small bunch basil
- 1 garlic clove
- 50g Brazil nuts, chopped
- juice of 1 lemon
- 25g Parmesan, grated (or vegetarian alternative)
- 2 tbsp rapeseed oil

Pop the watercress, basil, garlic and Brazil nuts into a food processor. Blitz until very finely chopped. Add the remaining pesto ingredients and pulse again until mixed, then season to taste. Serve stirred through pasta or spiralized courgetti, or with fish or chicken. Will keep, well covered, for 4–5 days in the fridge.

Nutrition: *per tbsp*
kcal 41 fat 4g saturates 1g carbs 0g sugars 0g fibre 0g protein 1g salt 0g

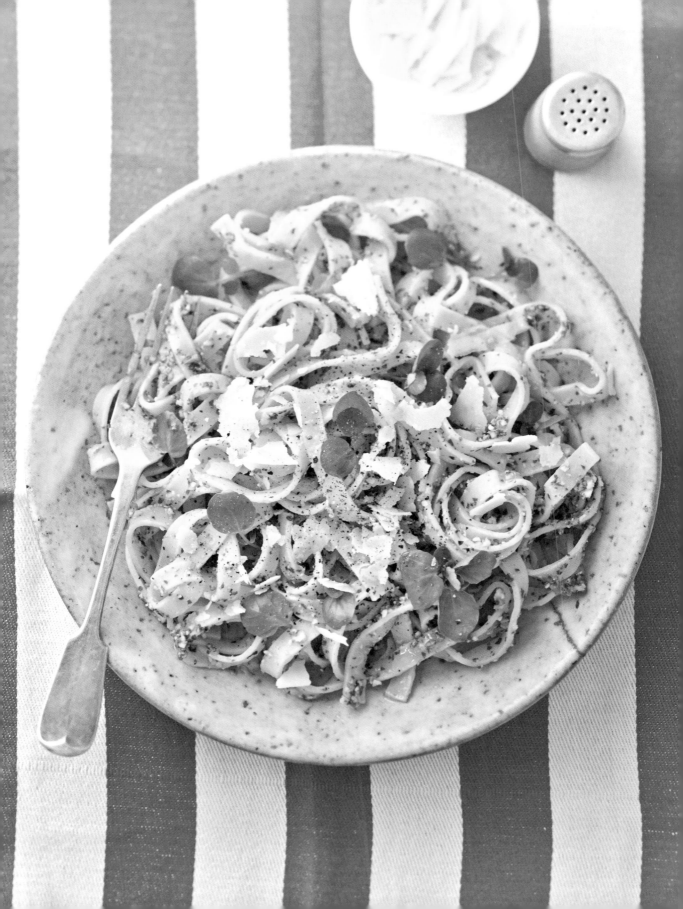

Ham & watercress salad with clementine dressing

Look for mixed whole-grain as opposed to 'white grains', which have had their nutrients stripped away. Quinoa, bulghar wheat and spelt are all good options.

🕐 PREP 20 mins NO COOK 🥧 4

- 250g pouch ready-to-eat mixed grains
- 280g leftover ham, shredded or cut into chunks
- 150g bag watercress
- 1 small fennel bulb, thinly sliced
- 50g hazelnuts, toasted and roughly chopped
- small bunch parsley, roughly chopped
- 1½ tbsp dried cranberries, roughly chopped

FOR THE DRESSING
- 2 tbsp extra virgin olive oil
- zest 1 clementine and juice of 2
- 2½ tsp Dijon mustard
- good drizzle of clear honey

1 For the dressing, put all the ingredients in a jar, along with some seasoning, pop on the lid and give it a really good shake.
2 Tip the grains into a large bowl and toss through the ham, watercress, fennel, hazelnuts and parsley. Just before serving, pour over the dressing and gently toss to combine. Transfer to a serving platter and scatter over the dried cranberries.

Nutrition: *per serving*
kcal 380 fat 18g saturates 2g carbs 27g sugars 10g fibre 9g protein 22g salt 1.8g

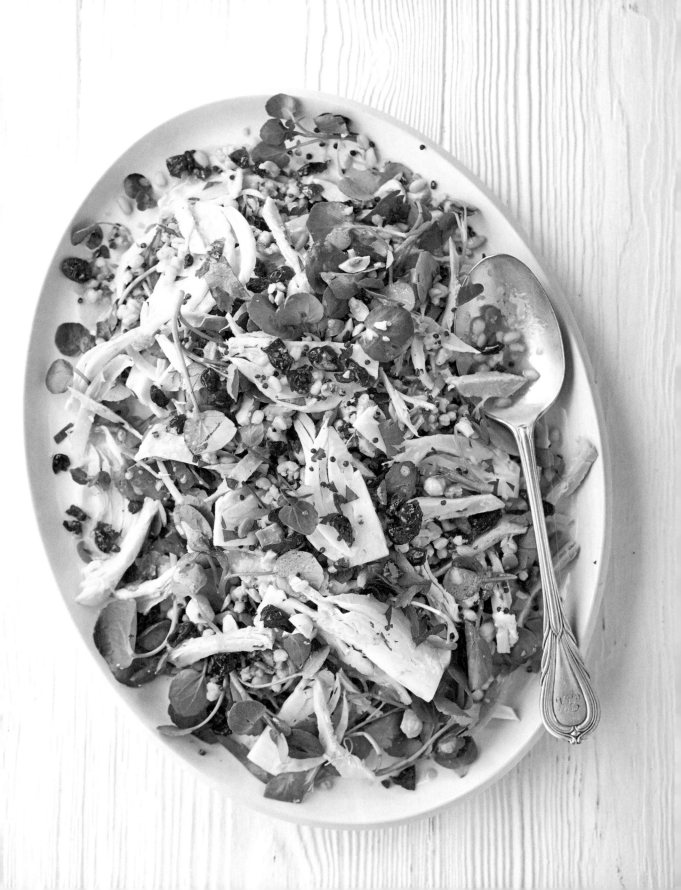

Purple sprouting broccoli with poached eggs & hollandaise

Purple sprouting broccoli contain all the nutrients of regular thin stemmed broccoli, and is nice to use when it's in season. This makes for an indulgent breakfast.

PREP 5 mins COOK 10 mins 2

- 250g purple sprouting broccoli
- 200g butter
- 6 medium eggs
- 1 tsp Dijon mustard
- 1 tbsp lemon juice
- a good pinch of chilli powder or a dash of Tabasco
- 2 slices sourdough bread

1 Cut any tough parts from the broccoli and cook the trimmed stems in boiling, lightly salted water for 3–4 mins. Drain and keep warm in a low oven along with 2 plates.

2 Next, make the sauce. Gently melt the butter in a small pan over a low heat. Meanwhile, crack 2 of the eggs into the jug of a blender and add the mustard, lemon juice and seasoning with a dash of chilli or Tabasco. Turn up the heat until the butter begins to bubble. With the motor running, pour it, in a thin stream, into the blender through the hole in the lid. Continue to run the motor for about 30 secs after all the butter is in to make sure the sauce is fully mixed. Set aside.

3 Heat a large pan of water. Crack an egg into a teacup and, once the water is simmering, tip the egg into the pan, then repeat with the 3 remaining eggs. Cook for 3 mins, then take them out in the order you put them in.

4 Meanwhile, toast the bread and keep warm. To serve, lay a slice of toast on each warm plate. Lift the eggs from the water using a slotted spoon, drain them well and place 2 eggs on each slice of toast. Serve the broccoli alongside and spoon some hollandaise sauce over, putting the rest in a small bowl. Serve at once.

Nutrition: *per serving*
kcal 564 fat 34g saturates 17g carbs 36g sugars 2g fibre 5g protein 24g salt 1.9g

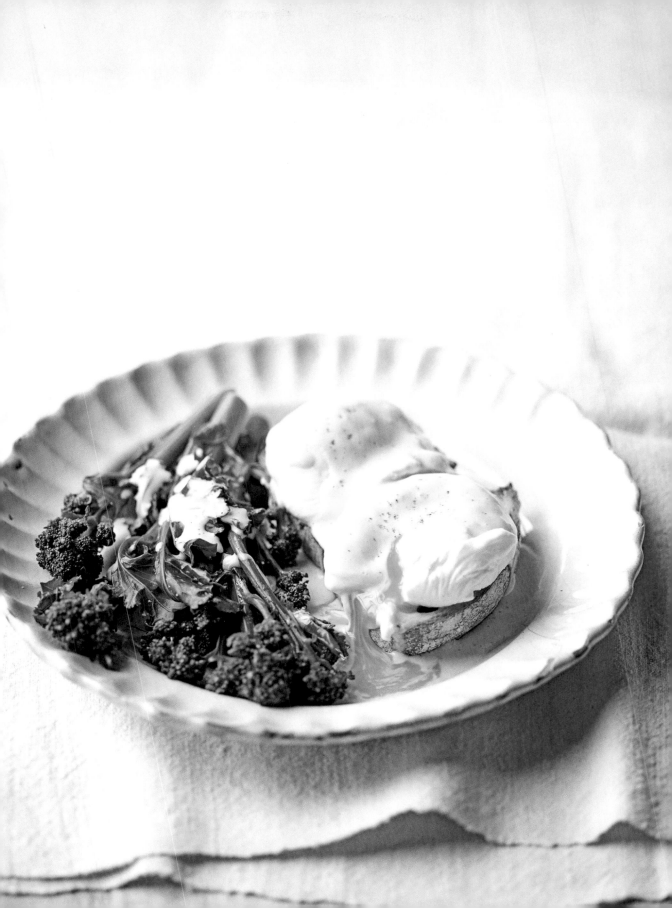

Green breakfast smoothie

Whizz up a green smoothie for breakfast, it's an easy way to start the day the right way.

🕐 PREP 10 mins NO COOK 🥧 2

- 1 handful spinach (about 50g), roughly chopped
- 100g broccoli florets, roughly chopped
- 2 celery sticks
- 4 tbsp desiccated coconut
- 1 banana
- 300ml rice or nut milk
- ¼ tsp spirulina (optional)

Whizz 300ml water and the ingredients in a blender until smooth.

Nutrition: *per serving*
kcal 243 fat 10g saturates 7g carbs 27g sugars 18g fibre 6g protein 7g salt 0.4g

Blackberry & beetroot smoothie

This purple smoothie has a hidden ingredient, kale! The sweet and spicy cinnamon and ginger will mask the earthy flavour, making for a delicious breakfast smoothie.

🕐 PREP 5 mins NO COOK 🥧 1

- 250ml coconut water
- pinch of ground cinnamon
- ¼ tsp ground nutmeg
- 4cm piece fresh ginger, peeled
- 1 tbsp shelled hemp seeds
- 2 small cooked beetroot, roughly chopped
- generous handful blackberries
- 1 pear, roughly chopped
- small handful kale

Add the coconut water to your blender with the spices and fresh ginger. Tip in the remaining ingredients and blend until smooth. Add more liquid if you prefer a thinner consistency. Pour into glasses and serve.

Nutrition: *per serving*
kcal 238 fat 6g saturates 1g carbs 37g sugars 34g fibre 8g protein 5g salt 0.3g

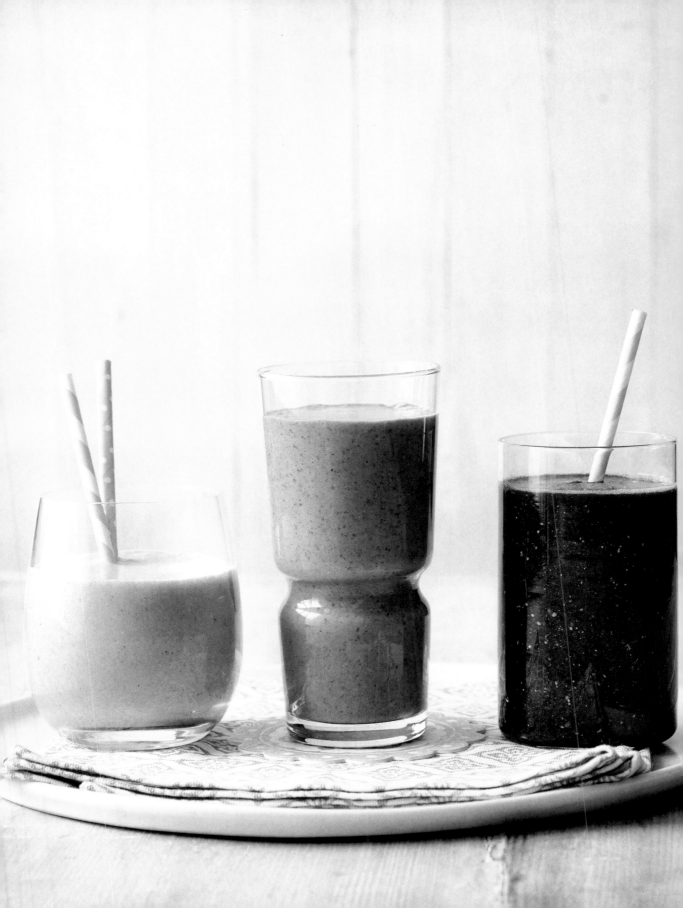

Chicken, broccoli & beet salad with avocado pesto

This superfood supper is packed with ingredients to give your body a boost, such as red onion, nigella seeds, walnuts, rapeseed oil and lemon.

PREP 15 mins COOK 15 mins 4

- 250g thin-stemmed broccoli
- 2 tsp rapeseed oil
- 3 skinless chicken breasts
- 1 red onion, thinly sliced
- 100g bag watercress
- 2 raw beetroots (about 175g), peeled and julienned or grated
- 1 tsp nigella seeds

FOR THE AVOCADO PESTO
- small pack basil
- 1 avocado, peeled and stoned
- ½ garlic clove, crushed
- 25g walnut halves, crumbled
- 1 tbsp extra virgin rapeseed oil
- juice and zest 1 lemon

1 Bring a large pan of water to the boil, add the broccoli and cook for 2 mins. Drain, then refresh under cold water. Heat a griddle pan, toss the broccoli in ½ tsp of the rapeseed oil and griddle for 2–3 mins, turning, until a little charred. Set aside to cool. Brush the chicken with the remaining oil and season. Griddle for 3–4 mins each side or until cooked through. Leave to cool, then slice or shred into chunky pieces.

2 Next, make the pesto. Pick the leaves from the basil and set aside a handful to top the salad. Put the rest in the small bowl of a food processor. Scoop the flesh from the avocado and add to the food processor with the garlic, walnuts, oil, 1 tbsp lemon juice, 2–3 tbsp cold water and some seasoning. Blitz until smooth, then transfer to a small serving dish. Pour the remaining lemon juice over the sliced onions and leave for a few mins.

3 Pile the watercress onto a large platter. Toss through the broccoli and onion, along with the lemon juice they were soaked in. Top with the beetroot, but don't mix it in, and the chicken. Scatter over the reserved basil leaves, the lemon zest and nigella seeds, then serve with the avocado pesto.

Nutrition: *per serving*
kcal 320 fat 18g saturates 3g carbs 8g sugars 6g fibre 6g protein 29g salt 0.3g

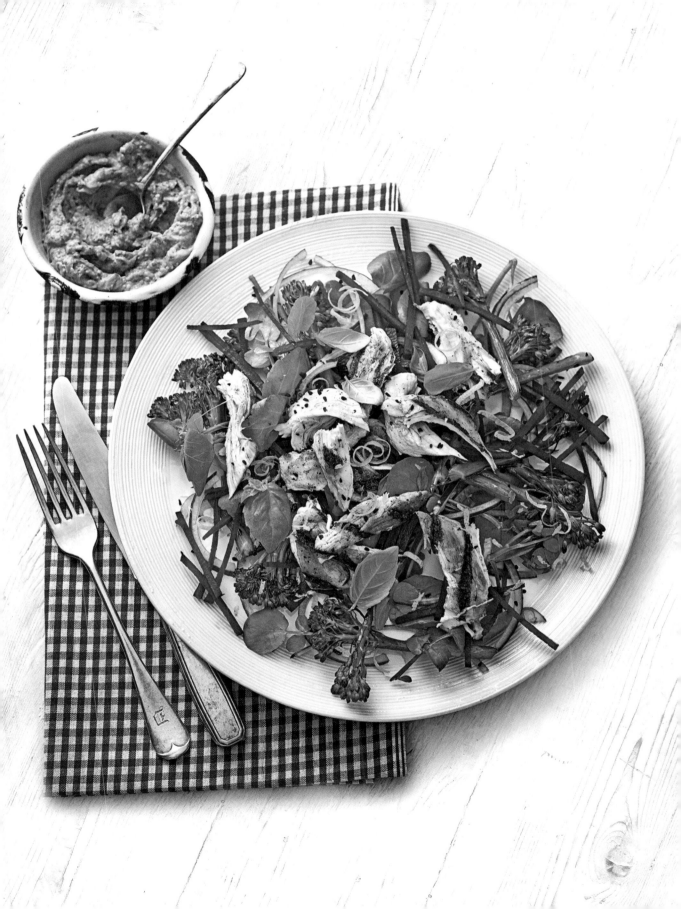

Superfood salad with citrus dressing

A quinoa salad packed full of the good stuff – broccoli, soya beans, avocados, spinach, herbs, pomegranate and pumpkin seeds.

PREP 25 mins COOK 5 mins 6

- 250g purple sprouting broccoli, cut in half (or into bite-sized chunks)
- 175g frozen soya beans or edamame
- 2 ripe avocados
- 250g pouch cooked quinoa
- 100g bag baby spinach
- handful soft herbs (parsley, basil, coriander or mint all work well), chopped
- 100g tub pomegranate seeds
- 100g bag pumpkin seeds, toasted in a dry pan until they pop

FOR THE CITRUS DRESSING
- zest and juice 1 lemon or lime
- zest and juice 1 orange
- 1 tbsp white wine vinegar
- 2 tbsp Dijon mustard
- 2 tbsp extra virgin rapeseed oil

1 Bring a saucepan of water to the boil and fill a large bowl with ice-cold water. Add the broccoli to the pan and cook for 2 mins, then add the soya beans and cook for 1–2 mins more until the broccoli is cooked but still has a bite. Drain and drop the vegetables straight into the cold water – this quickly cools them, retaining their bite and bright colour. Leave for 1–2 mins until cool, then drain and leave in the colander while you prepare the remaining ingredients.

2 Dry the large bowl. Add the dressing ingredients with some seasoning and whisk together. Halve, stone and peel the avocados, then cut into chunky dice and add straight to the dressing (this will stop the avocado turning brown). Add the quinoa, spinach, herbs, half the pomegranate and pumpkin seeds, and the cooked vegetables to the bowl, and gently toss everything together. Transfer the salad to a serving platter, scatter with the remaining seeds and serve. Any leftovers will keep in the fridge for lunch the next day.

Nutrition: *per serving*
kcal 349 fat 23g saturates 3g carbs 22g sugars 6g fibre 8g protein 13g salt 0.9g

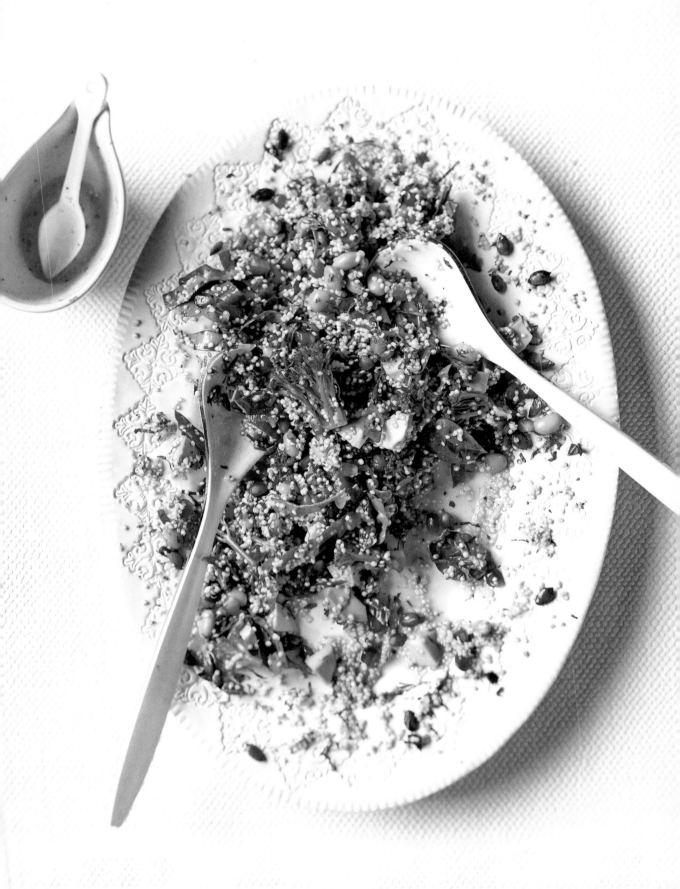

Kale, tomatoes & poached eggs on toast

Kale is full of the good stuff, but can be a little tough. Remove the woody stalks before chopping to make it a little less fibrous.

PREP 2 mins COOK 7 mins 2

- 2 tsp oil
- 150g kale, chopped
- 1 garlic clove, crushed
- ½ tsp chilli flakes
- 2 large eggs
- 2 slices multigrain bread
- 50g cherry tomatoes, halved
- 15g feta, crumbled

1 Bring a large pan of water to the boil. Heat the oil in a frying pan over a medium heat and add the kale, garlic and chilli flakes. Cook, stirring occasionally, for 4 mins until the kale begins to crisp and wilt to half its size. Set aside.
2 Adjust the heat so the water is at a rolling boil, then poach your eggs for 2 mins. Meanwhile, toast the bread.
3 Remove the poached eggs with a slotted spoon and top each piece of toast with half the kale, an egg, the cherry tomatoes and feta.

Nutrition: *per serving*
kcal 315 fat 16g saturates 4g carbs 19g sugars 3g fibre 5g protein 19g salt 0.8g

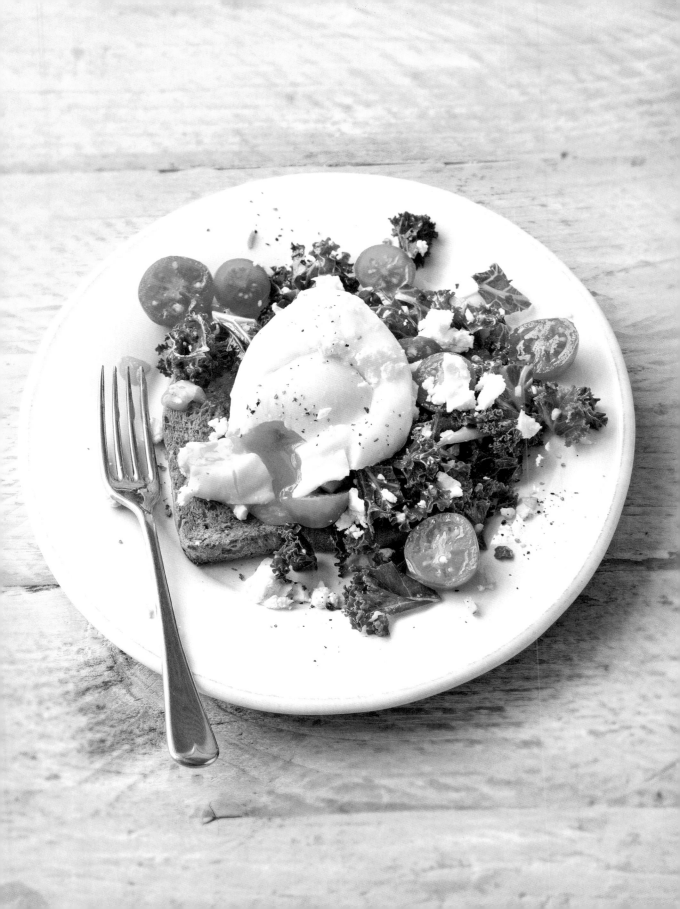

Green goddess smoothie bowl

Smoothies aren't just for drinking. Smoothie bowls are thicker than a regular smoothie, so you can top it with nutrient dense toppings such as seeds and fruit.

PREP 15 mins COOK 15 mins plus freezing · 2

- 2 bananas, sliced
- 1 ripe avocado, stoned, peeled and chopped into chunks
- 1 small ripe mango, stoned, peeled and chopped into chunks
- 150g spinach (fresh or frozen)
- 250ml milk (unsweetened almond or coconut milk works well)
- 1 tbsp unsweetened almond or peanut butter
- 1 tbsp clear honey, agave or maple syrup (optional)

FOR THE SEED MIX
- 1 tbsp chia seeds
- 1 tbsp linseeds
- 4 tbsp pumpkin seeds
- 4 tbsp sunflower seeds
- 4 tbsp coconut flakes
- 4 tbsp flaked almonds
- ¼ tsp ground cinnamon
- 2 tbsp clear honey, agave or maple syrup

FOR THE TOPPING
- 175g mixed fresh fruit, chopped (we used banana, mango, raspberries and blueberries)

1 Slice the bananas and arrange over a small baking tray lined with parchment. Freeze for 2 hrs until solid. (You can now transfer the banana slices to a freezer bag and freeze for 3 months, or continue with the recipe.)

2 For the seed mix, heat oven to 180C/160C fan/gas 4 and line a baking tray with parchment. Tip the seeds, coconut and almonds into a bowl, add the cinnamon and drizzle over the honey, agave or maple syrup. Toss until everything is well coated, then scatter over the baking tray in an even layer. Bake for 10–15 mins, stirring every 5 mins or so, until the seeds are lightly toasted. Leave to cool. Will keep in an airtight container for up to 1 month.

3 Put the avocado, mango, spinach, milk, nut butter, frozen banana slices and honey (if using) in a blender and whizz to a thick smoothie consistency – you may have to scrape down the sides with a spoon a few times. Divide between two bowls and arrange the fruit on top. Scatter 1–2 tbsp of the seed mix over each bowl and eat straight away.

Nutrition: *per serving*
kcal 493 fat 24g saturates 5g carbs 52g sugars 48g fibre 12g protein 11g salt 0.2g

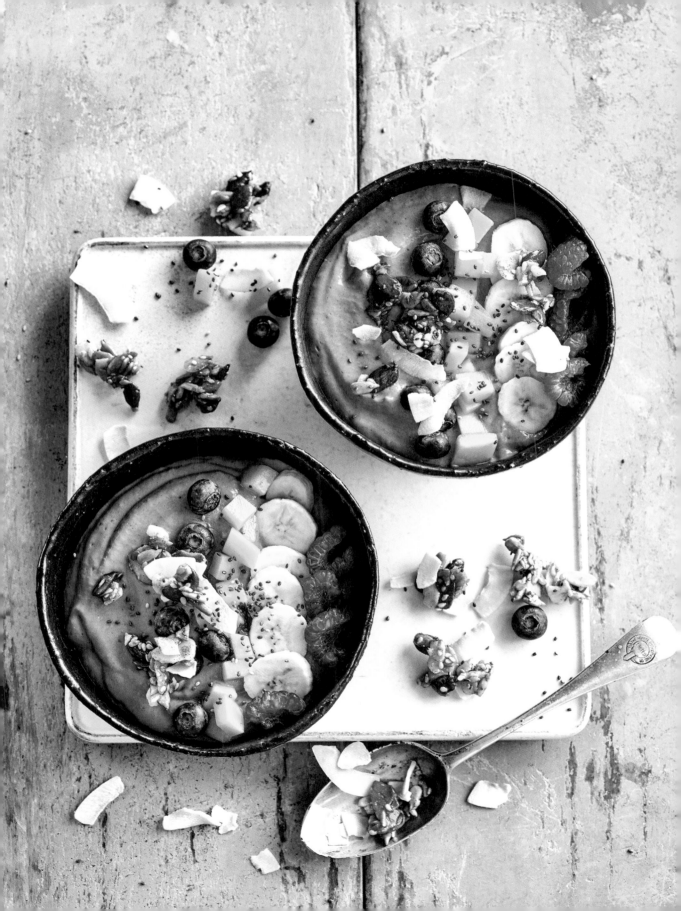

Spinach & sweet potato samosas

These samosas freeze really well. Assemble them, then wrap in clingfilm and freeze for up to 3 months. Cook from frozen, adding an extra 5–10 mins to the cooking time.

PREP 35 mins COOK 45 mins 3

- 2 large sweet potatoes (about 500g), peeled and cut into small pieces
- 1 tbsp vegetable oil, plus extra for brushing
- 2 red onions, 1 chopped, 1 halved and finely sliced
- thumb-sized piece ginger, peeled and finely chopped
- 2 garlic cloves, crushed
- 1 fat red chilli, finely chopped (optional)
- small bunch coriander, stalks finely chopped, leaves picked
- 2 tbsp curry paste (we used balti)
- 2 tsp black onion (nigella) seeds
- 300g spinach (or frozen spinach)
- 270g pack filo pastry (6 sheets)
- ½ cucumber
- 150ml pot natural yogurt
- mango chutney, to serve

1 Put the sweet potatoes in a large bowl, cover with cling film and microwave on High for 8 mins or until soft.

2 Meanwhile, heat the oil in a large pan, add the chopped onion and cook for a few mins to soften. Stir in the ginger, garlic, chilli (if using) and coriander stalks, stirring for a couple mins more until fragrant (the garlic will burn easily, so keep an eye on it). Add the curry paste and half the black onion seeds to the pan, stir for 30 secs or so until fragrant, then add the spinach and 2–3 tbsp water. Cook the spinach until wilted, then add the sweet potato and any liquid from the bowl. Season well and mash everything together with the back of a spoon, leaving some chunky bits of potato. Leave to cool completely.

3 Unroll the pastry and pull out 2 sheets to work with – keep the rest covered with a tea towel to prevent it from drying out. Brush both sheets with a little oil and scatter some of the black onion seeds over one sheet. Put the other sheet on top. With the shortest side facing you, cut down the centre to make 2 long strips. Scoop a sixth of the sweet potato mixture onto the top right-hand corner of the filo in a rough triangle shape. Fold the pastry over on an angle, continuing down the length of the pastry until you reach the bottom and have a neat triangle encasing the filling. Trim off any excess pastry with a knife. Repeat to make 6 samosas. Heat oven to 200C/180C fan/gas 6.

4 Put the samosas on a baking tray lined with baking parchment. Brush with a little more oil and sprinkle over the remaining black onion seeds. Bake for 25–30 mins or until deep golden brown. Meanwhile, peel the cucumber into ribbons, then toss with the sliced onions and coriander leaves. To serve, dollop some yogurt onto each plate, top with two samosas, a mound of the cucumber salad and mango chutney.

Nutrition: *per serving*
kcal 659 fat 13g saturates 2g carbs 108g sugars 36g fibre 15g protein 18g salt 1.5g

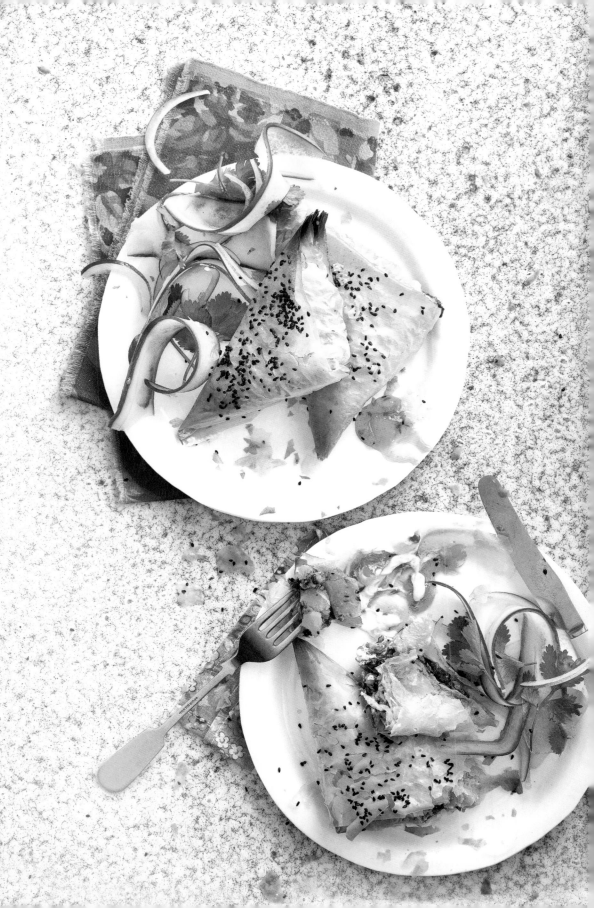

Fried egg Florentine toastie

We've served this toastie with sriracha hot sauce, it's super-spicy so if you prefer leave it out or replace it with milder sweet chilli sauce.

PREP 10 mins COOK 10 mins 1

- 2 slices of white bread
- knob of butter
- 25g cheddar, grated
- handful baby spinach
- 1 tbsp olive oil
- 1 medium egg
- sriracha hot sauce, to serve
- extra spinach or watercress, to serve

1 Remove the centre of both slices of bread with the rim of a drinking glass or a cookie cutter. Spread each slice with a little butter and top both with the cheddar and torn spinach leaves – pack as much cheese and spinach on as you can. Heat a large non-stick pan over a medium heat and drizzle in the oil.

2 Once the pan is hot, sandwich the bread together. Using a fish slice, place in the pan and press down to brown. Cook for 4–5 mins on a medium heat until the cheese begins to melt.

3 Flip the sandwich over and crack the egg into the hole in the middle. Cover the pan with a lid to cook the egg through for 3–4 mins. Transfer to a plate, drizzle over some sriracha and serve with spinach or watercress on the side.

Nutrition: *per serving*
kcal 480 fat 34g saturates 12g carbs 22g sugars 2g fibre 2g protein 20g salt 1.3g

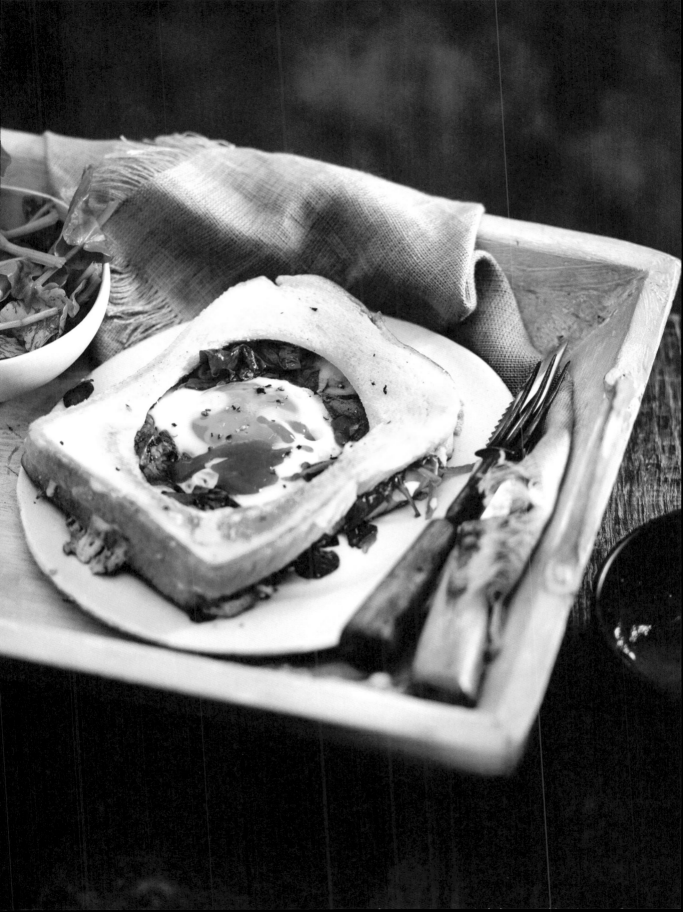

Fresh raspberry jelly

Who says superfoods have to come in salad form? Get your intake of red berries with this zingy dessert. You can also use frozen raspberries if fresh ones aren't in season.

PREP 15 mins plus setting COOK 10 mins   4

- ½ tsp flavourless oil for greasing, such as sunflower oil
- 5 gelatine leaves
- 140g golden caster sugar
- 500g raspberries, plus extra to serve
- juice 1 lemon
- clotted cream or ice cream, to serve

1 Use the oil to lightly grease the inside of a 600ml jelly mould. Put the gelatine leaves in a small bowl of cold water, one at a time so they don't stick together. Leave to soak while you cook the raspberries.

2 Pour 300ml water into a large saucepan. Add the caster sugar, heat gently over a medium heat, stirring occasionally until the sugar has dissolved, then add the raspberries. Bring to the boil, then turn the heat right down so the mixture is barely simmering, and cook for 5 mins until the raspberries break down. Stir well, but don't mash them too much as the raspberries will break down in the heat.

3 Carefully pour the raspberry mixture through a sieve set over a large heatproof measuring jug. Stir in the lemon juice, then either top up with cold water or pour some away to ensure you have exactly 600ml total liquid. Drain the water from the gelatine leaves and squeeze out any excess before adding to the raspberry mix. Stir well until the gelatine has completely dissolved, then pour into your jelly mould. Once cold, place in the fridge and leave overnight to set.

4 Turn the jelly out onto a large plate just before serving. Serve with a scoop of clotted cream or ice cream, and some raspberries.

Nutrition: *per serving*
kcal 191 fat 1g saturates 0g carbs 41g sugars 41g fibre 4g protein 3g salt 0g

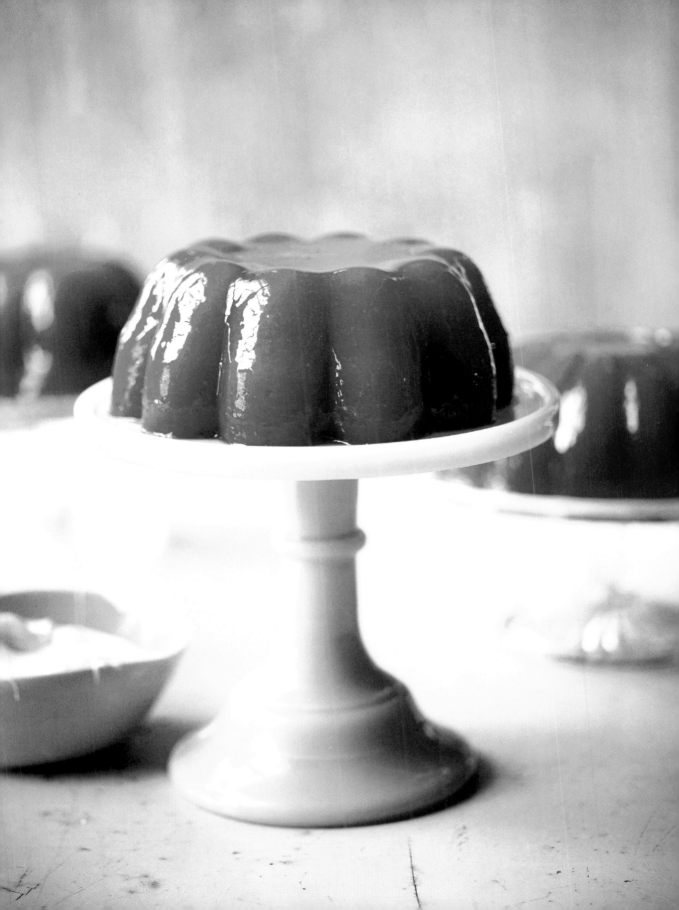

Coconut crêpes with raspberry sauce

This raspberry sauce would also be nice served with thick Greek yogurt and granola.

PREP 10 mins COOK 25 mins 6

FOR THE RASPBERRY SAUCE
- 300g raspberries
- 2 tsp cornflour
- 2 tsp maple syrup

FOR THE COCONUT CRÊPES
- 140g plain flour
- 2 large eggs
- 300ml coconut milk
- 2 tbsp toasted desiccated coconut
- a little sunflower oil, for frying

1 Set aside 6 of the raspberries. Mix the cornflour with 1 tbsp water until smooth. Measure 300ml water in a pan, and stir in the cornflour paste. Heat, stirring, until thickened. Add the remaining raspberries and cook gently, mashing the berries to a pulp. Strain the mixture through a sieve into a bowl to remove the seeds, pushing through as much of the mixture as you can. Quarter the reserved raspberries and add to the sauce, along with the maple syrup.

2 To make the crêpes, tip the flour and a pinch of salt into a large jug, then beat in the eggs, coconut milk, 200ml water and 1½ tbsp toasted coconut to make a batter the consistency of double cream. Thin with a little more water if it is too thick. Heat a small frying pan with a dash of oil, then pour in a little batter, swirling the pan so that it completely covers the base. Leave to set over the heat for 1 min, then carefully flip it over and cook the other side for a few secs more. Transfer to a plate and repeat with the remaining batter until you have at least 12. Stir the batter to redistribute the coconut as you use it. Serve 2 crêpes per person with a drizzle of the sauce and a little of the remaining toasted coconut.

Nutrition: *per serving*
kcal 258 fat 14g saturates 11g carbs 25g sugars 5g fibre 4g protein 6g salt 0.1g

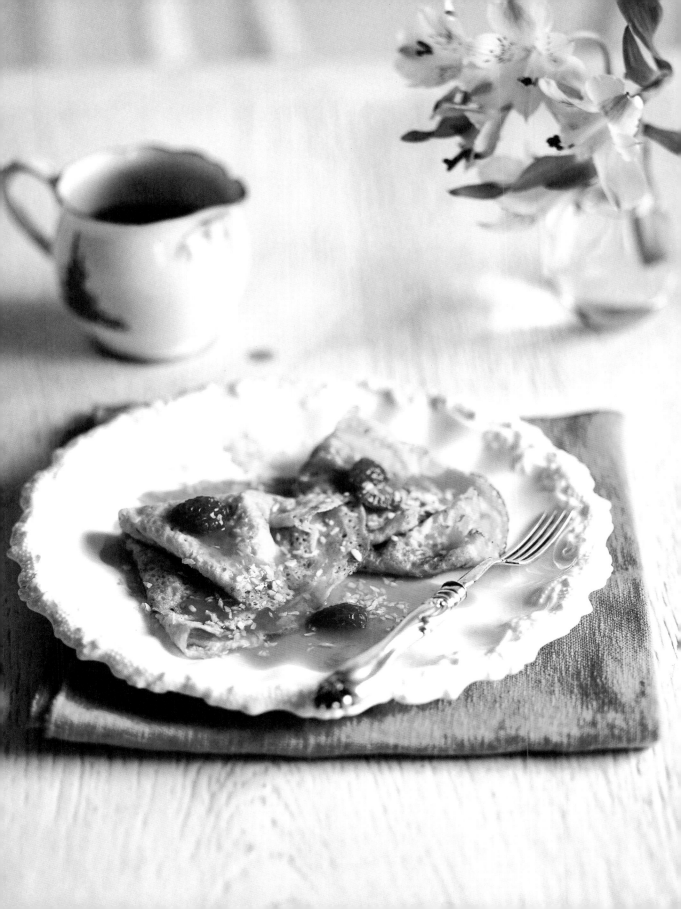

Strawberry & watermelon slushie

Kids will love this refreshing fruit slushie. You could also freeze the mixture in lolly moulds for an icy treat.

🕐 PREP 10 mins NO COOK 🍽 6

- 1 small watermelon
- 225g punnet of ripe strawberries, tops cut off
- juice of 2 limes

1 The day or morning before you want to drink the slushie cut the watermelon into chunks and remove the skin and seeds. Place half the watermelon wedges into a large freezable bag then pop in the freezer for a few hours.
2 Once frozen, blitz the frozen watermelon with the rest of the watermelon, strawberries and lime juice until smooth and slushy. Pour into glasses and sip through a straw.

Nutrition: *per serving*
kcal 142 fat 1g saturates 0.4g carbs 29g sugars 29g fibre 2g protein 2g salt 0g

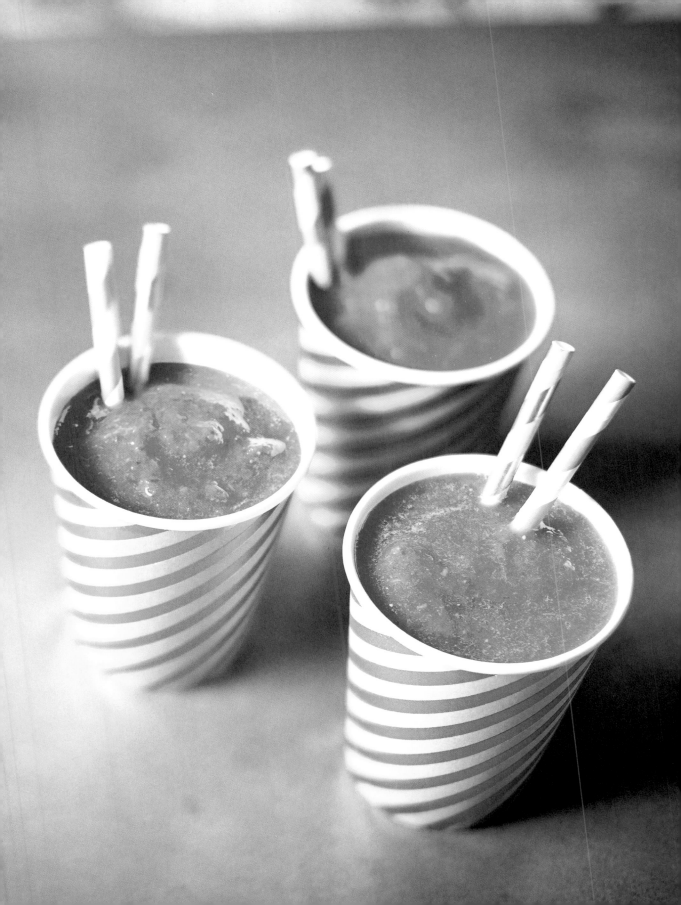

Spiced salmon with beetroot, feta & wild rice

Ready-cooked beetroot is a convenient ingredient to keep in your fridge. It keeps for weeks and can be transformed into dinner in a dash.

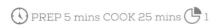 PREP 5 mins COOK 25 mins 1

- 1 salmon fillet
- ¼ tsp ground cumin
- ¼ tsp caraway seeds
- 1 tsp extra virgin olive oil, plus extra to serve
- 60g wild rice
- 100g ready-cooked beetroot, cut any way you like
- 2 spring onions, sliced on a diagonal
- juice ½ lemon
- 25g feta, roughly crumbled

1 Before you prep the veg, coat the salmon fillet in the spices and oil then set aside to marinate. In a small saucepan with a tight-fitting lid simmer the rice over a medium heat for 25 mins.

2 After 15 mins, season the salmon, then place the fish, skin-side down, in a cold non-stick frying pan (this will ensure you get an evenly crispy skin). Place over a medium-high heat and cook the salmon for 5 mins, then flip it over and cook on the other side for 1–2 mins more, depending on how you like it.

3 Drain the rice, then return it to the saucepan and toss with the beetroot, spring onions, lemon juice and seasoning to taste. Serve the rice alongside the spiced salmon with the crumbled feta and a drizzle of olive oil on top.

Nutrition: *per serving*
kcal 626 fat 27g saturates 7g carbs 53g sugars 9g fibre 6g protein 39g salt 1g

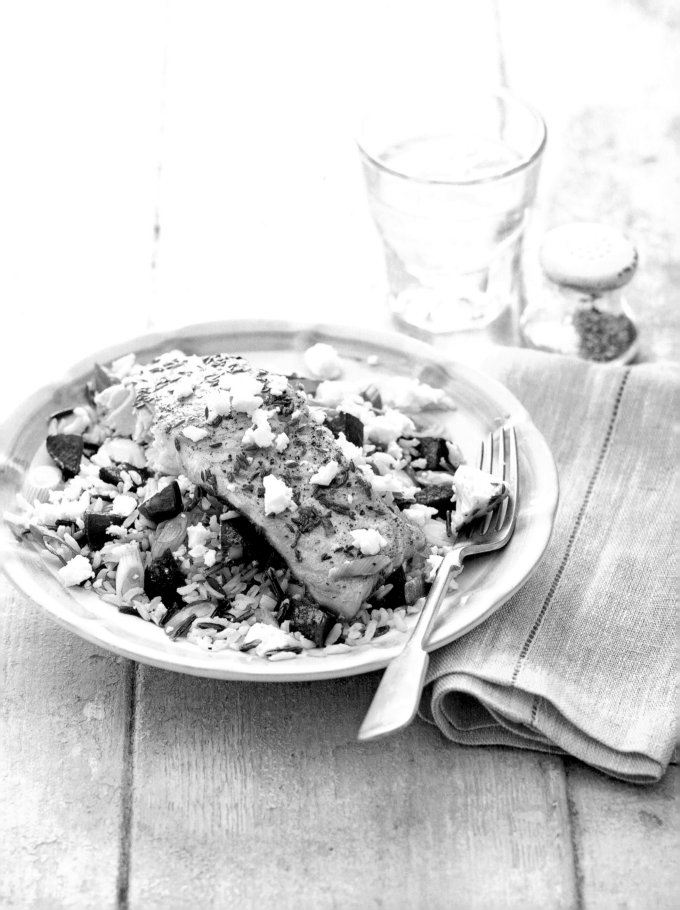

Trout with tomato sauce

Canned tomatoes are preserved in tins when they're at their peak, meaning for most of the year they have a better flavour than their fresh counterparts. Cooking tomatoes helps to increase their levels of lycopene, a powerful antioxidant.

PREP 5 mins COOK 25 mins 2

- 1½ tbsp olive oil
- 1 shallot, thinly sliced
- 2 garlic cloves, crushed
- 1 bay leaf
- 400g can chopped tomatoes
- 1 tsp sherry vinegar
- 1 tbsp butter
- 2 rainbow trout fillets, pin-boned, skin left on (if the fillets are large, cut in half lengthways or ask your fishmonger to do this for you)
- handful mixed olives, stones removed
- handful basil, shredded
- good-quality extra-virgin olive oil, for drizzling

1 In a frying pan, heat 1 tbsp of oil over a low-medium heat. Add the shallot and a pinch of salt, then cook, stirring occasionally, for 8 mins until softened and the edges begin to brown. Stir in the garlic and cook for 1 min, then add the bay leaf, tomatoes, vinegar and seasoning. Stir well, bring to the boil, then reduce the heat and simmer gently for 15 mins.

2 After the sauce has been simmering for 7 mins, heat the remaining oil with the butter in a non-stick frying pan over a medium-high heat. Season the fish well and place, skin-side down, in the pan. Cook for 4 mins – try not to move the fish so the skin gets evenly coloured. Flip over and continue to cook for 2 mins or until the flesh begins to flake in large chunks.

3 Season the sauce to taste, then spoon some onto each plate and top with a fillet. Scatter over the olives and the basil, then drizzle over the extra virgin olive oil to serve.

Nutrition: *per serving*
kcal 429 fat 25g saturates 8g carbs 9g sugars 8g fibre 2g protein 40g salt 0.9g

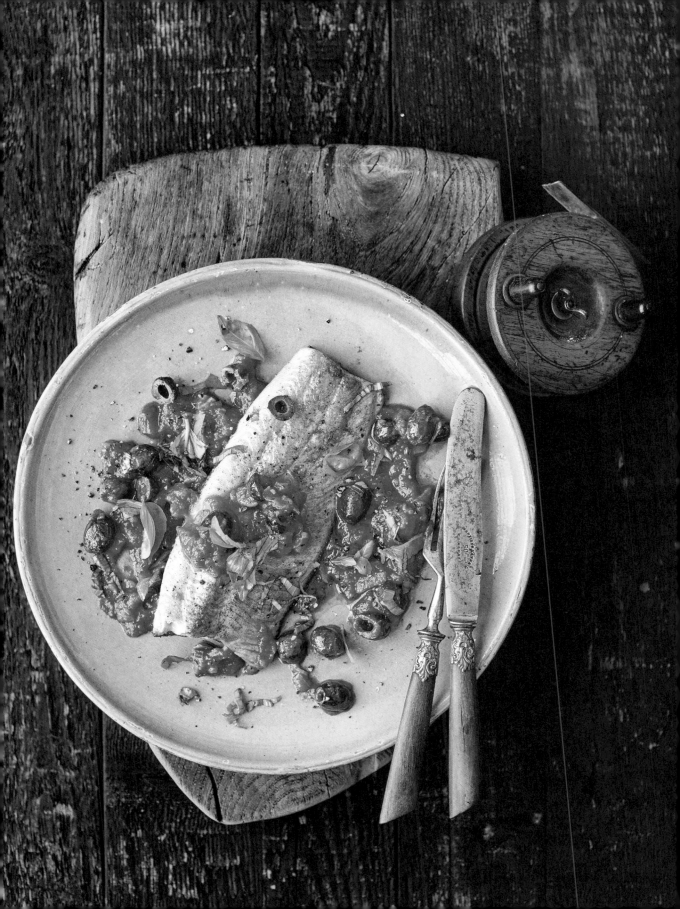

Beetroot & onion seed soup

A deep red soup that's low fat, vegetarian and full of flavour. Beetroot and apple give this soup a subtle sweet flavour, while lentils add protein and bulk

🕐 PREP 5 mins COOK 5 mins 🥧 1

- 250g cooked beetroot
- 100g canned lentils
- 1 small apple
- 1 crushed garlic clove
- 1 tsp onion seeds (nigella), plus extra to serve
- 250ml vegetable stock

Tip the beetroot, lentils, apple, garlic and onion seeds into a blender with the vegetable stock and some seasoning, and blitz until smooth. Heat until piping hot in the microwave or on the hob, then scatter over some extra onion seeds, if you like.

Nutrition: *per serving*
kcal 257 fat 2g saturates 0g carbs 41g sugars 30g fibre 10g protein 12g salt 1.2g

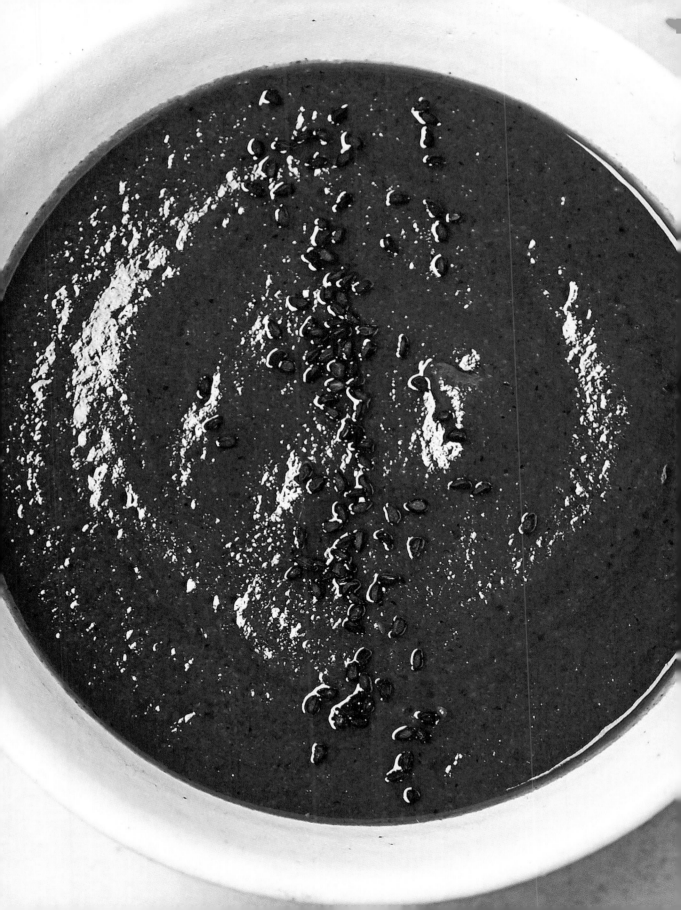

Warm beet, chorizo & pear salad

This is a great dinner party dish. Look out for rainbow beetroots when they're in season. Candy striped and golden varieties look nice.

PREP 15 mins COOK 55 mins | 4

- 1kg mixed beets, leaves trimmed
- 200g chorizo, skinned skinned and sliced
- 100g whole blanched almonds
- 2 tbsp membrillo (quince paste)
- 4 tbsp Sherry vinegar
- 1 tbsp lemon juice, plus an extra squeeze
- 1 tbsp extra virgin olive oil
- 1 large pear or 2 small firm pears (I used Red Williams)
- small pack parsley, leaves picked and roughly torn
- 50g Manchego, shaved

1 Put the beets in a large pan of water (if you have a mix of colours, cook in separate pans as the colours will bleed). Bring the water to a boil, cover and leave to simmer – about 20–40 mins, depending on the size of the beets. Use a skewer or small sharp knife to check that they're tender in the centre (try not to poke too often or they'll bleed all their juices into the water).

2 Drain the beets and leave to cool in a colander. When cool enough to handle, peel away the skins, root and stalks, then roughly chop or slice the beets.

3 Put the chorizo in a cold frying pan and fry over a medium heat until crisp – you should collect lots of oil in the pan. Lift out the chorizo with a slotted spoon and keep warm. Tip in the almonds and fry quickly until just turning brown on the edges. Scoop out with a slotted spoon and place on kitchen paper to dry.

4 Make the dressing by melting the membrillo in the pan with the chorizo oil, Sherry vinegar and 1 tbsp lemon juice. Mix in the olive oil and season. Core and thinly slice the pear, toss with a little lemon juice to stop it browning, then arrange on a platter with the beets, chorizo and almonds.

5 Toss together with the dressing, if you like, or serve the dressing on the side. Sprinkle over the parsley and Manchego and serve immediately.

Nutrition: *per serving*
kcal 568 fat 33g saturates 10g carbs 37g sugars 34g fibre 9g protein 24g salt 1.7g

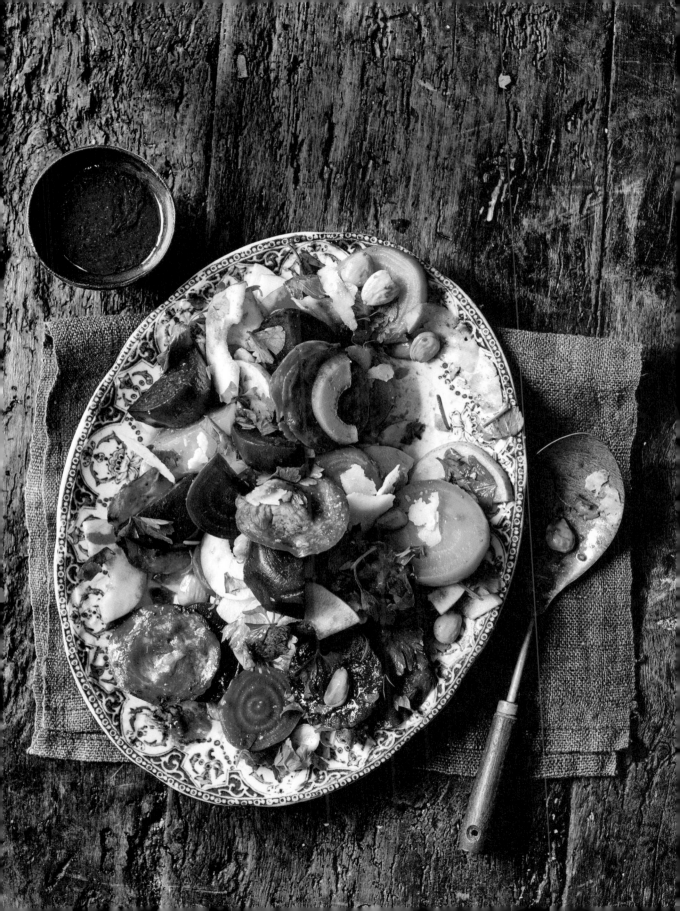

Baked sweet potato with lentils & red cabbage slaw

This simple vegetarian main course is rich in calcium and iron, and comes with a vibrant, crunchy coleslaw to really make your plate pop!

PREP 20 mins COOK 40 mins   2

- 2 sweet potatoes (about 175g), washed and patted dry
- 1 tbsp extra virgin rapeseed oil
- 1 medium onion, finely sliced
- 2 garlic cloves, crushed
- thumb-sized piece ginger, peeled and finely grated
- 1 long green chilli, finely chopped (deseeded if you don't like it too hot)
- 2 tsp ground cumin
- 2 tsp ground coriander
- 85g split red lentils
- finely grated zest ½ lemon, plus 2 tbsp juice
- 2 medium-large tomatoes, roughly chopped
- ½ small pack coriander, roughly chopped, plus a few sprigs to garnish
- 4 tbsp full-fat plain bio-yogurt
- lemon wedges, for squeezing over (optional)

FOR THE RED CABBAGE SLAW
- 2 tbsp extra virgin olive oil
- 2 tsp lemon juice
- ¼ small red cabbage, cored and very finely sliced
- 1 medium carrot, peeled and coarsely grated
- 2 spring onions, finely sliced
- 25g sultanas
- 1 tbsp mixed seeds, such as sunflower, pumpkin, sesame and linseed

1 Heat oven to 220C/200C fan/gas 7. Put the sweet potatoes on a baking tray and bake for 40 mins or until soft. Meanwhile, heat the oil in large non-stick saucepan over a medium-high heat. Fry the onion for 3–5 mins or until pale golden brown, stirring constantly, making sure it doesn't burn. Add the garlic, ginger, chilli and spices, and cook for a few secs, stirring constantly.

2 Add the lentils to the pan, pour over 400ml water, stir well and bring to the boil. Skim off any foam that rises to surface with a spoon. Add ½ tsp flaked sea salt, the lemon zest and 1 tbsp of the lemon juice, stir well and reduce the heat to low.

3 Cover the pan loosely with a lid and leave to simmer gently for 20 mins or until the lentils are tender, stirring occasionally. Add the tomatoes, coriander and remaining 1 tbsp lemon juice, and cook for a further 5 mins, stirring. If the lentils thicken too much, add a splash of water. Season to taste.

4 To make the red cabbage slaw, whisk the oil and lemon juice together in a large bowl and season with lots of ground black pepper. Add the cabbage, carrot, spring onions, sultanas and seeds, then toss together well.

5 Put the potatoes on 2 plates, split them and fill with the lentils. Spoon over the yogurt, garnish with coriander and serve with the coleslaw and lemon wedges for squeezing over, if you like.

Nutrition: *per serving*
kcal 752 fat 24g saturates 4g carbs 100g sugars 53g fibre 17g protein 23g salt 1.8g

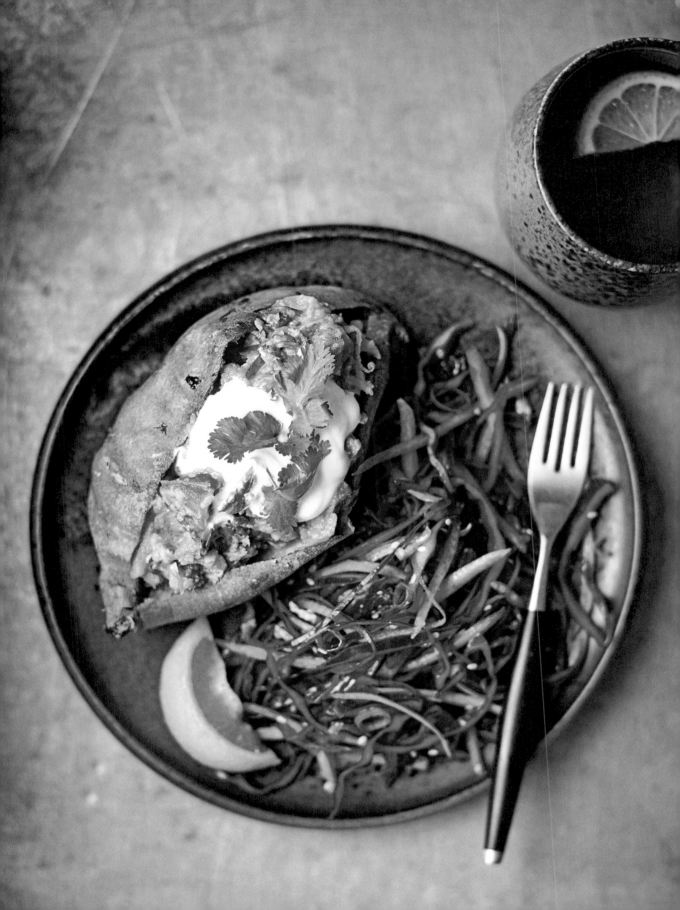

Halloumi & red cabbage steaks

Here's a new way to cook your cabbage! These roasted steaks have a wonderful nutty flavor.

PREP 15 mins COOK 40 mins 4

- 1 small red cabbage (about 900g), cut into 4 x 2cm thick 'steaks'
- 2 tbsp balsamic vinegar
- 2 tbsp olive oil
- 1 tsp fennel seeds
- 1 tbsp dark muscovado sugar
- 2 x 250g pouches ready-cooked quinoa
- juice 1 orange
- small pack flat-leaf parsley, chopped
- small pack dill, chopped
- 50g dried sour cherry, roughly chopped
- 250g pack halloumi, cut into 8 slices

1 Heat oven to 200C/180C fan/gas 6. Line a baking tray with baking parchment and put the cabbage steaks on top. Mix together the balsamic, oil, fennel seeds and sugar, then season and spoon it over the cabbage. Cover the cabbage with foil and roast for 20 mins, then remove the foil and cook for a further 10 mins until softened.

2 Heat the quinoa following pack instructions, then stir through the orange juice, parsley, dill and cherries, and season with black pepper. Fry the halloumi in a dry pan on a medium heat for 2 mins each side until golden. To serve, place a spoonful of quinoa onto each cabbage steak and top with the halloumi.

Nutrition: *per serving*
kcal 658 fat 30g saturates 12g carbs 66g sugars 24g fibre 11g protein 25g salt 3g

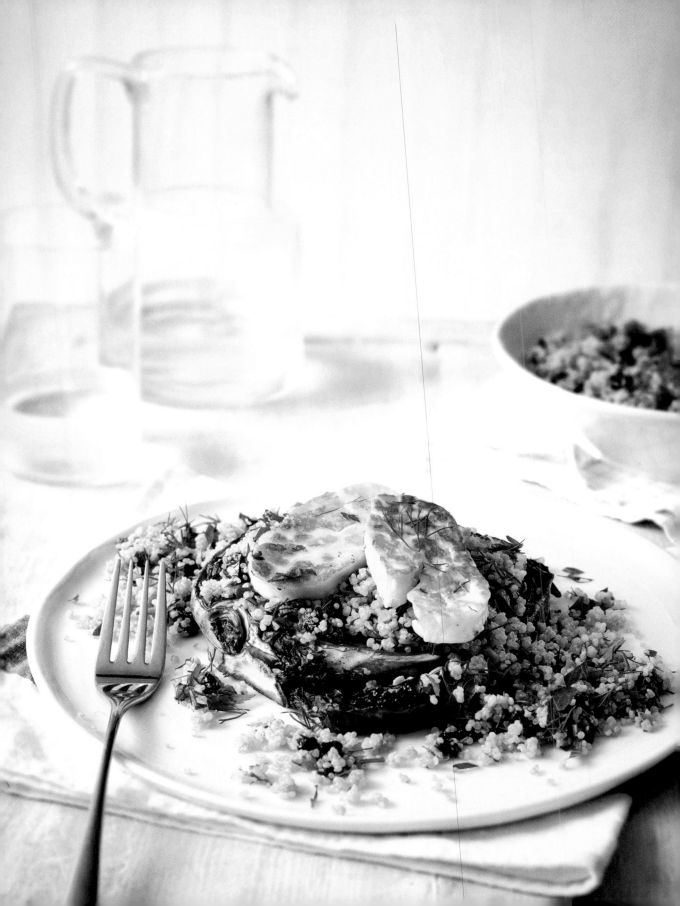

Crunchy red cabbage slaw

Serve this simple slaw with roast chicken pieces or with hotdogs.

🕐 PREP 15 mins NO COOK 🥧 4

- ½ red cabbage, shredded
- 2 tbsp sesame seeds
- 2 tbsp pumpkin seeds
- 2 tbsp sunflower oil
- 1 tbsp red wine vinegar
- 2 tsp soy sauce
- 1 tsp golden caster sugar

1 Put the red cabbage in a large bowl with the seeds and toss to combine.
2 Make the dressing by mixing all the remaining ingredients together in a small bowl or jug. Pour the dressing over the cabbage and seeds, and serve immediately.

Nutrition: *per serving*
kcal 157 fat 11g saturates 2g carbs 8g sugars 5g fibre 3g protein 4g salt 0.5g

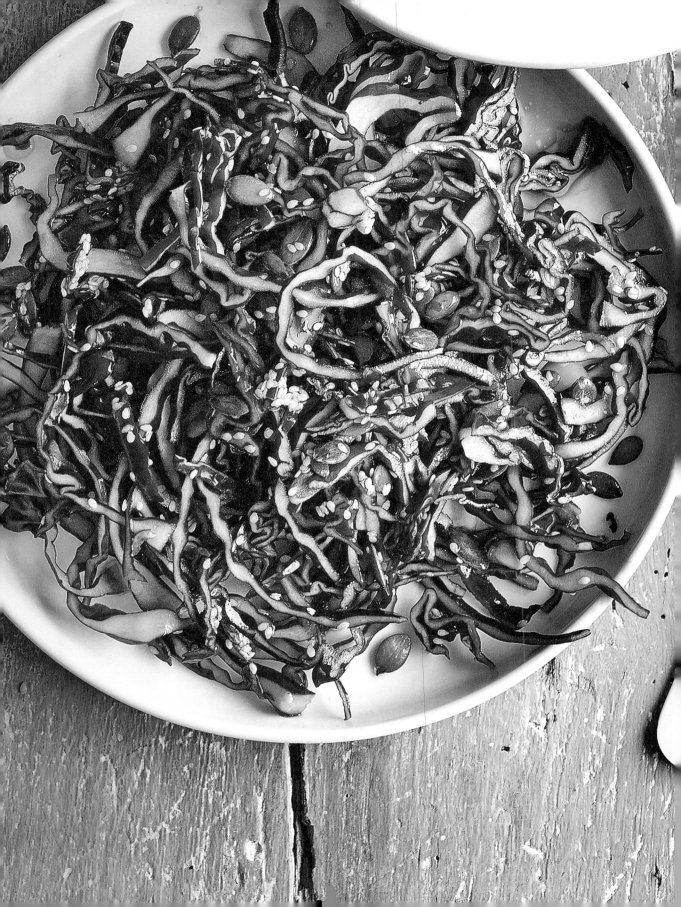

Hot'n'spicy tomato & red pepper soup

This vibrant soup is packed with antioxidants and lycopene, and can be on the table in under 10 mins.

PREP 3 mins COOK 5 mins 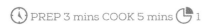 1

- 290g roasted red peppers, drained
- 270g cherry tomatoes, halved
- 1 garlic clove, crushed
- 1 vegetable stock cube
- 1 tsp paprika
- 1 tbsp olive oil
- 4 tbsp ground almonds

Put the roasted red peppers in a blender with the cherry tomatoes, garlic, vegetable stock cube, 100ml water, paprika, olive oil and ground almonds. Blitz until smooth, season well and heat until piping hot before serving.

Nutrition: *per serving*
kcal 631 fat 48g saturates 5g carbs 23g sugars 12g fibre 5g protein 23g salt 3g

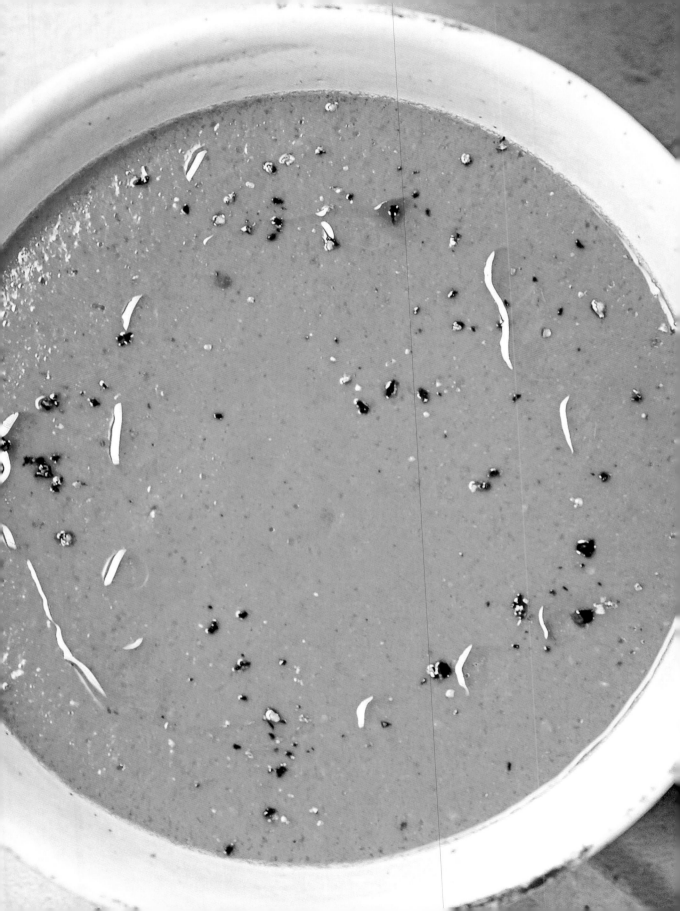

Smoky shakshuka

Shakshuka is a popular Middle-Eastern dish of eggs baked in a spicy tomato based sauce. This simple version includes chorizo for an extra smoky flavour.

PREP 5 mins COOK 15 mins 2

- ½ a ring of chorizo
- 2 roasted red peppers, from a jar
- 1 can chopped tomatoes
- 2 eggs

1 Slice the chorizo and cook in a frying pan until the oils are released. Slice the peppers, add to the pan with the tomatoes, season and cook until warmed through.
2 Make 2 spaces in the pan and crack an egg into each one. Cover with a lid and simmer for 5 mins until the eggs are cooked.

Nutrition: *per serving*
kcal 348 fat 23g saturates 8g carbs 11g sugars 8g fibre 2g protein 23g salt 2.2g

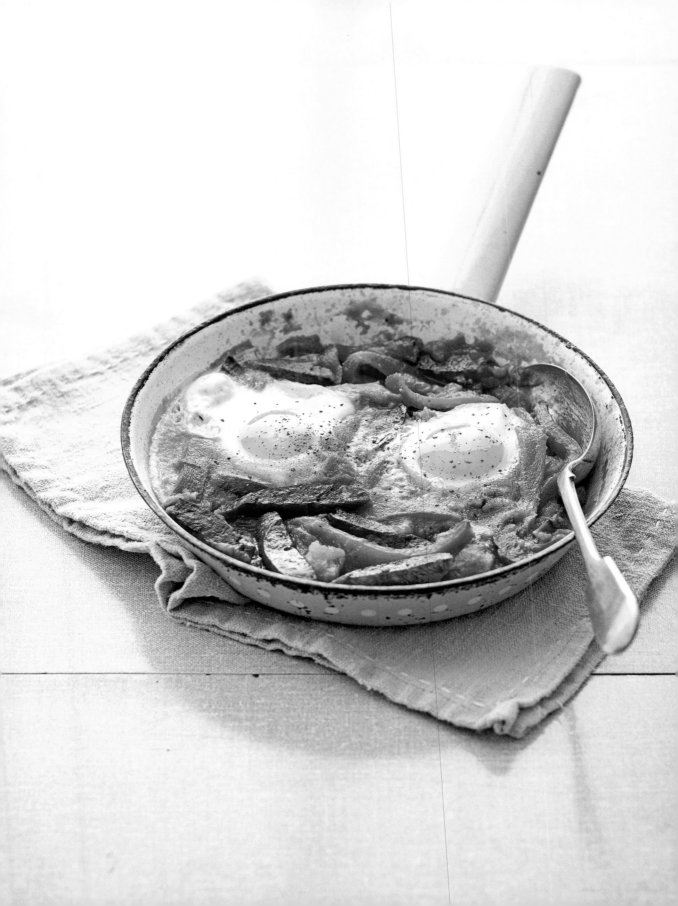

Omelette pancakes with tomato & pepper sauce

A quick, light supper, perfect for those busy days when you want something simple to eat.

🕐 PREP 10 mins COOK 20 mins 🥧 2

- 4 large eggs
- handful basil leaves

FOR THE SAUCE
- 2 tsp extra virgin rapeseed oil plus a little extra for the pancakes
- 1 yellow pepper, quartered, deseeded and thinly sliced
- 2 garlic cloves, thinly sliced
- 1 tbsp cider vinegar
- 400g can chopped tomatoes
- wholemeal bread or salad leaves, to serve

1 First make the sauce. Heat the oil in a large frying pan, and fry the pepper and garlic for 5 mins to soften them. Spoon in the cider vinegar and allow to sizzle away. Tip in the tomatoes, then measure in a third of a can of water. Cover and leave to simmer for 10–15 mins until the peppers are tender and the sauce is thick.

2 Meanwhile, make the pancakes. Beat 1 egg with 1 tsp water and seasoning, then heat a small non-stick frying pan with a tiny amount of oil. Add the egg mixture and cook for 1–2 mins until set into a thin pancake. Lift onto a plate, cover with foil and repeat with the other eggs. Roll up onto warm plates, spoon over the sauce and scatter with the basil. Serve with bread or a salad on the side.

Nutrition: *per serving*
kcal 271 fat 17g saturates 3g carbs 11g sugars 10g fibre 4g protein 16g salt 0.6g

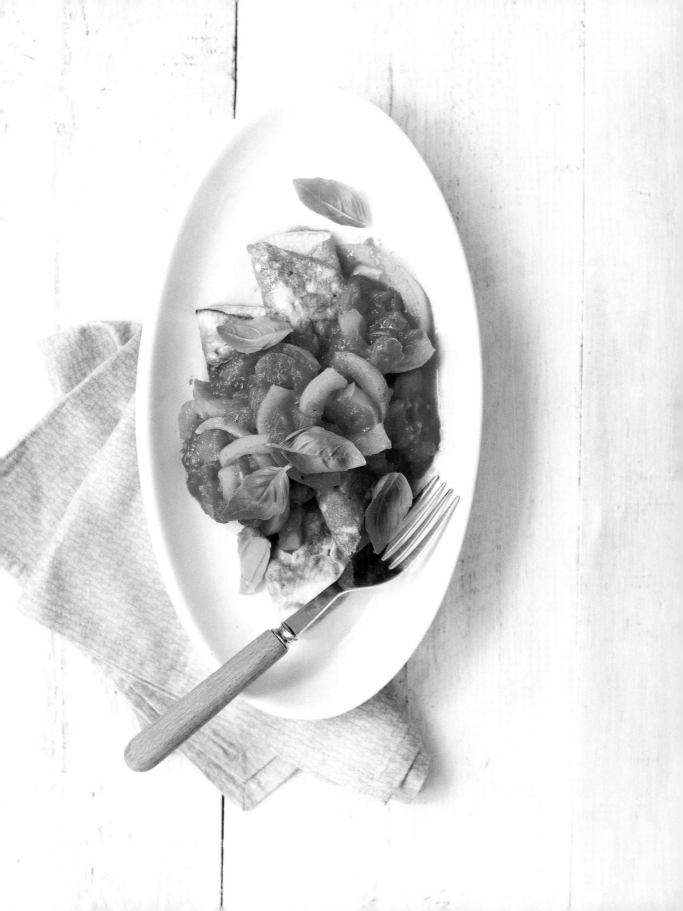

Tomato & courgette risotto

You can replace the risotto rice with wholegrain pearl barley if you want to boost the nutrients in this dish.

PREP 10 mins COOK 30 mins | 2

- 2 tbsp olive oil
- 1 small onion, diced
- 2 garlic cloves, crushed
- ½ tsp coriander seeds, crushed
- 200g risotto rice
- 500ml vegetable stock
- 200g carton passata
- 12 cherry tomatoes, halved
- 2 courgettes, halved and sliced
- 2 tbsp mascarpone
- Parmesan (or vegetarian alternative), grated, to serve

1 Put 1 tbsp of oil in a large pan over a medium heat. Add the onion and cook for 5–7 mins until softened. Add the garlic and coriander seeds and cook, stirring, for another 1 min. Stir in the risotto rice, coating it in the onion mixture. Gradually add 300ml of the vegetable stock, stirring until fully absorbed by the rice between each addition. Pour the passata into the risotto, cover and simmer for 10–15 mins. Stir occasionally and add more stock as needed.

2 Meanwhile, heat oven to 200C/180C fan/gas 6. Put the cherry tomatoes and courgettes in a roasting tin, keeping them separate, drizzle with 1 tbsp olive oil, season and roast for 10–12 mins until just tender.

3 Add the mascarpone and plenty of seasoning to the risotto. Stir until the rice is completely cooked and the risotto is creamy, about 5 mins more. Add the courgettes and stir to combine. Serve the risotto in bowls topped with the roasted tomatoes and some grated Parmesan.

Nutrition: *per serving*
kcal 633 fat 23g saturates 8g carbs 90g sugars 13g fibre 6g protein 13g salt 0.7g

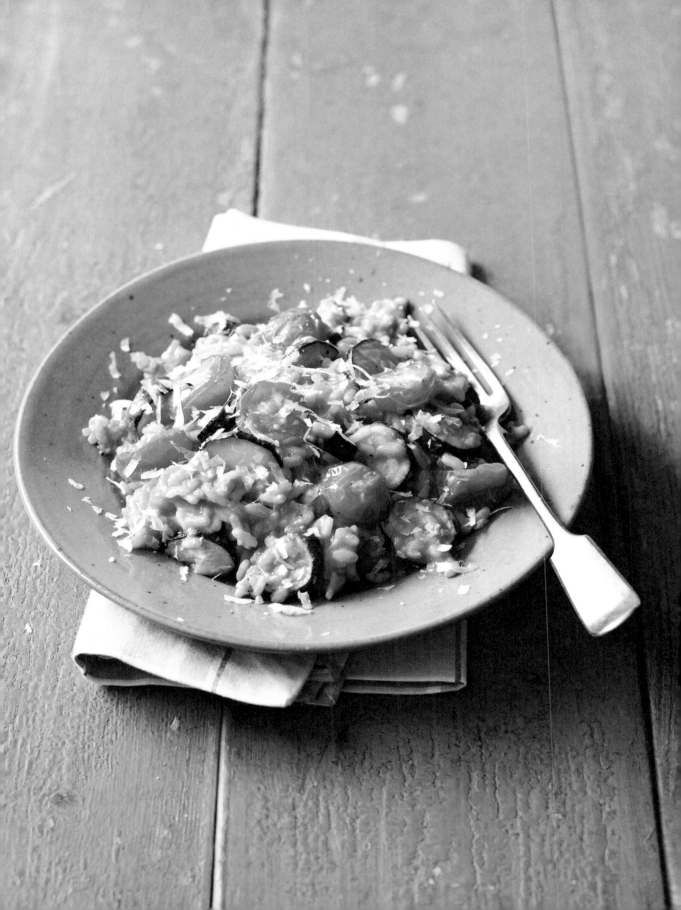

Orange & blueberry bircher

Bircher is a healthy breakfast dish of oats soaked in water, milk or apple juice. Chill overnight and top with fresh, seasonal fruit.

PREP 5 mins plus soaking overnight NO COOK ⟅ 2

- 70g porridge oats
- 2 tbsp golden linseeds
- zest of ½ orange, plus 2 peeled and chopped oranges
- 175g tub natural yogurt
- 150g blueberries

1 Mix the oats and golden linseeds with the zest of ½ an orange. Pour over 300ml boiling water and leave overnight.

2 The next day, stir in three-quarters of a 175g tub of yogurt, spoon into glasses or bowls, top with 2 peeled and chopped oranges, the remaining yogurt and the blueberries.

Nutrition: *per serving*
kcal 345 fat 9g saturates 3g carbs 48g sugars 22g fibre 8g protein 13g salt 0.2g

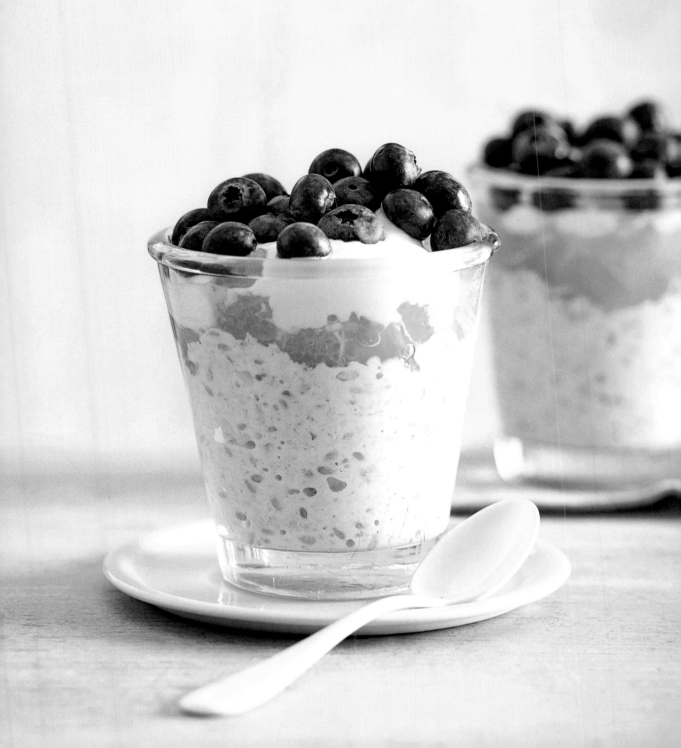

Citrus salmon salad

Fresh and zingy citrus fruit cuts through the richness of salmon in this speedy dish.

PREP 2 mins COOK 8 mins 2

- 2 salmon fillets
- 1 large grapefruit
- 2 tbsp extra virgin olive oil
- 100g bag watercress
- 100g feta, crumbled

1 Heat oven to 200C/180C fan/ gas 6 and roast the salmon for 8 mins. Meanwhile, segment the grapefruit and mix the juices with the extra virgin olive oil to make a dressing.
2 Toss the watercress with the grapefruit segments, dressing and feta, and serve with the salmon, flaked into large pieces.

Nutrition: *per serving*
kcal 570 fat 43g saturates 12g carbs 6g sugars 6g fibre 3g protein 39g salt 1.5g

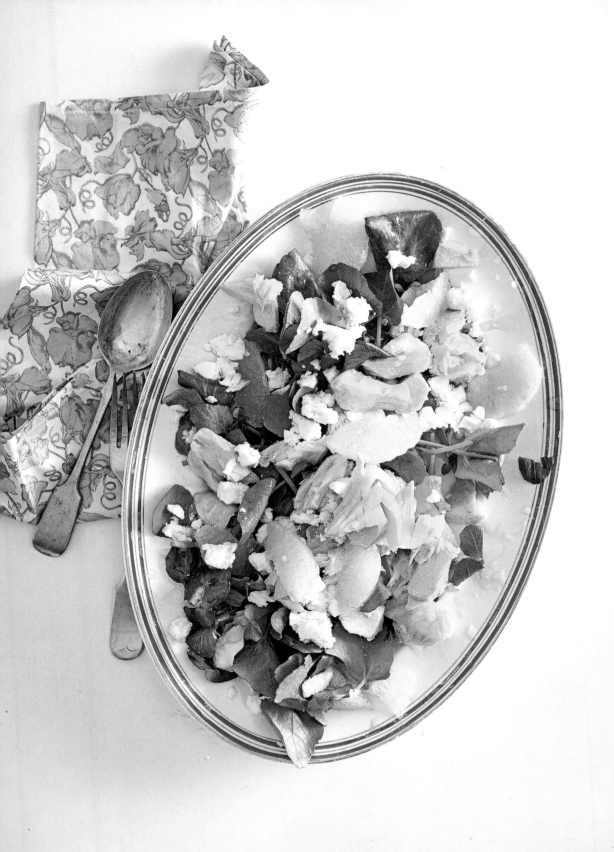

Winter squash, apple & kale panzanella

This winter version of the classic panzanella salad uses roasted squash and kale in place of the usual tomatoes.

PREP 20 mins COOK 40 mins · 4

- ½ large butternut squash, cut into chunks
- 4 tbsp extra virgin olive oil
- 6 sage leaves, chopped
- 2 apples, cored and sliced into slim wedges
- 3 tbsp clear honey, plus extra for drizzling
- 200g leftover crusty bread (we used ciabatta), torn into chunks
- 100g hazelnuts, roughly chopped
- 4 tbsp red wine vinegar
- 200g bag chopped kale
- 100g dried cranberries

1 Heat oven to 200C/180C fan/gas 6. Put the squash on a baking tray, drizzle with 1 tbsp oil and scatter over the sage and some seasoning. Toss together, then bake for 30 mins.
2 Add the apple slices to the tray, drizzle over the honey and toss with the squash. Put the bread on a separate tray and return both trays to the oven. Bake for another 10–15 mins until the squash and apple are tender and starting to caramelise, and the bread is crisp. Meanwhile, toast the hazelnuts in a small pan until golden. Remove the trays from the oven and set aside to cool a little.
3 Whisk the remaining oil, the honey and vinegar in a large bowl with some seasoning. Add the kale, cranberries, hazelnuts, squash apples and toasted bread. Toss everything together, then transfer to a platter or plates to serve.

Nutrition: *per serving*
kcal 648 fat 30g saturates 3g carbs 77g sugars 42g fibre 9g protein 13g salt 0.8g

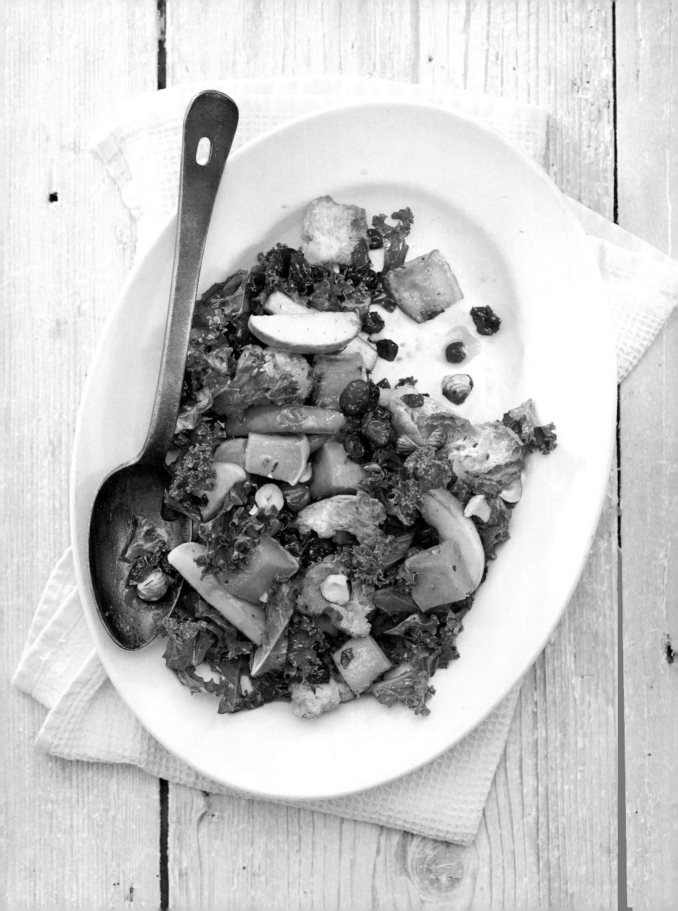

Sunshine lollies

If you don't have any lolly moulds, you can make these lollies in cleaned yogurt pots. Cover the tops with foil to hold the lolly stick in place whilst freezing.

PREP 20 mins plus freezing NO COOK 6

- 5 large carrots
- juice of 3 large oranges, zest of 1
- 1 satsuma, peeled then chopped (optional)

Finely grate the carrots and place in the middle of a clean tea towel. Gather up the towel, and squeeze the carrot juice into a jug, discarding the pulp. Add the orange juice and top up with a little cold water if needed to make up 360ml liquid. Stir in the orange zest and satsuma pieces, if using. Pour into lolly moulds and freeze overnight.

Nutrition: *per lolly*
kcal 17 fat 0g saturates 0g carbs 4g sugars 4g fibre 0g protein 0g salt 0g

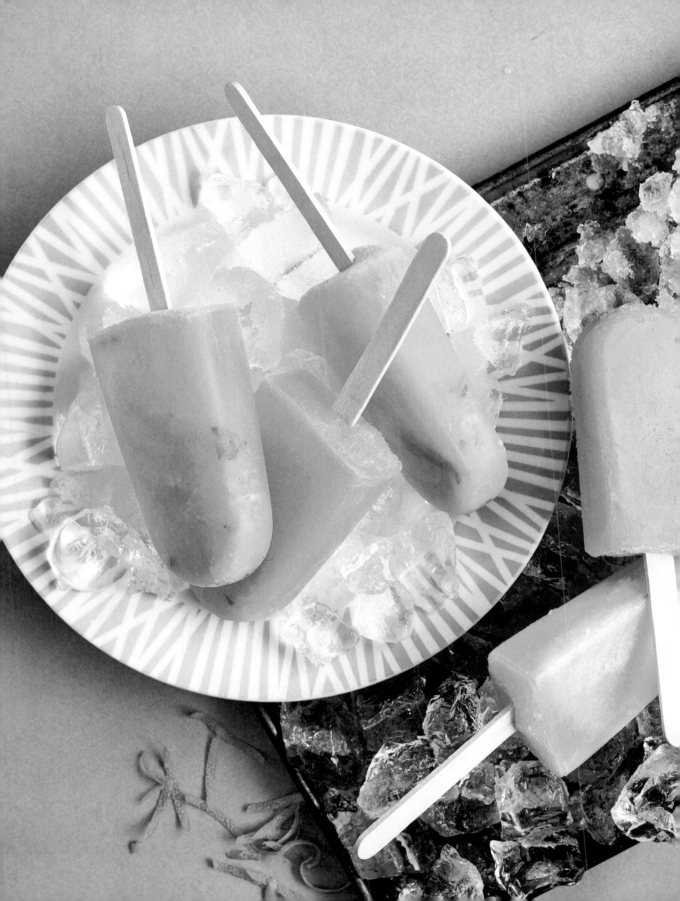

Orange, fennel & wild rice salad

Serve this salad on a big platter alongside a roast chicken or glazed ham.

⏱ PREP 45 mins COOK 25 mins 🥧 8

- 500g carrots (we used purple and orange ones), peeled, halved and cut into short batons on an angle
- 1 tbsp olive oil
- 100g mixed basmati & wild rice
- 75g Puy lentils
- 3 oranges
- large fennel bulb, quartered, core removed, thinly sliced
- 1 red onion, halved and thinly sliced
- 200g seedless red grapes, halved
- 100g pecans, chopped
- large handful parsley, chopped
- large handful mint, chopped

FOR THE DRESSING
- 2 tbsp Dijon mustard
- zest and juice 1 lemon
- 4 tbsp olive oil
- 1 tbsp maple syrup

1 Heat oven to 200C/180C fan/gas 6. Toss the carrots, oil and some seasoning on a large baking tray. Cook for 25–30 mins until tender. While the carrots cook, fill 2 large pans with salted water and bring to the boil. Add the rice to one pan and the lentils to the other. Cook following pack instructions, or until just cooked, then drain and set aside to cool.

2 Zest the oranges over a large bowl. Cut away the peel and pith, then cut along each piece of membrane to remove the segments, catching any juices in the bowl. Set the segments aside. Add the ingredients for the dressing to the orange zest and juice, season and whisk.

3 When the carrots have cooled a little, add to the dressing with the remaining salad ingredients, including the cooked rice, lentils and orange segments. Toss together and serve on a big platter.

Nutrition: *per serving*
kcal 332 fat 17g saturates 2g carbs 34g sugars 17g fibre 8g protein 7g salt 0.6g

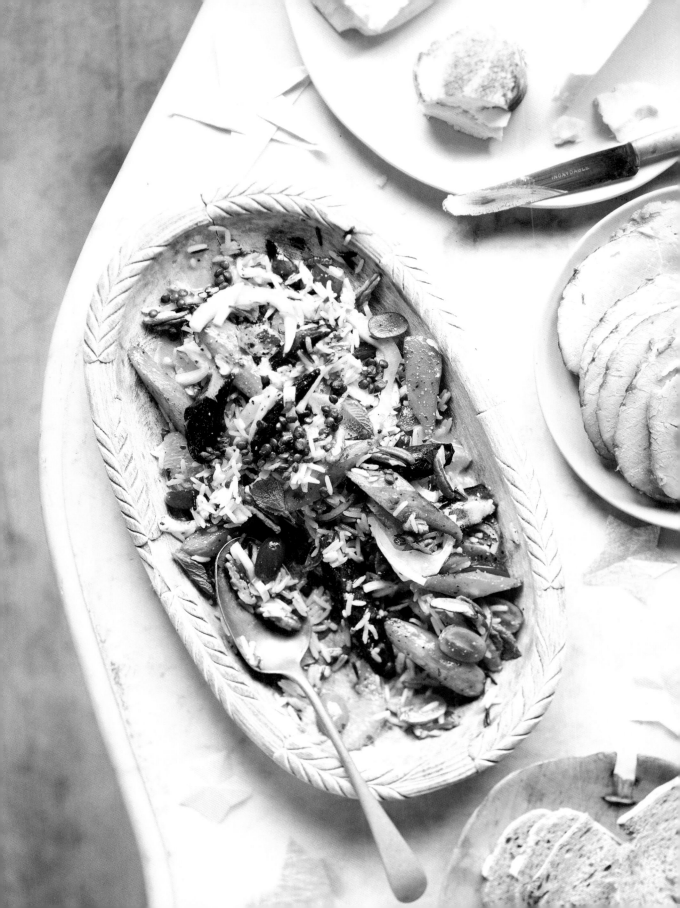

Orange & raspberry granola

Make your own oat milk in this recipe for no-added-sugar granola, or serve with organic cow's milk or yogurt.

PREP 15 mins plus chilling COOK 25 mins 4

- 400g jumbo oats
- juice 2 oranges (150ml), plus zest of ½
- 1 tsp ground cinnamon
- 2 tbsp freeze-dried raspberries or strawberries
- 25g flaked almonds, toasted
- 25g mixed seeds (such as sunflower, pumpkin, sesame and linseed)

TO SERVE
- 2 large oranges, peeled and segmented
- mint leaves (optional)

1 Put 200g oats and 500ml water in a food processor and blitz for 1 min. Line a sieve with clean muslin and pour in the oat mixture. Leave to drip through for 5 mins, then twist the ends of the muslin and squeeze well to capture as much of the oat milk as possible – it should be the consistency of single cream. Best chilled at least 1 hr before serving. Can be kept in a sealed or covered jug in the fridge for up to 3 days.

2 Heat oven to 200C/180C fan/gas 6 and line a baking tray with baking parchment. Put the orange juice in a medium saucepan and bring to the boil. Boil rapidly for 5 mins or until the liquid has reduced by half, stirring occasionally. Mix the remaining 200g oats with the orange zest and cinnamon. Remove the pan from the heat and stir the oat mixture into the juice. Spread over the lined tray in a thin layer and bake for 10–15 mins or until lightly browned and crisp, turning the oats every few mins. Leave to cool on the tray.

3 Once cool, mix the oats with the raspberries, flaked almonds and seeds. Can be kept in a sealed jar for up to one week. To serve, spoon the granola into bowls, pour over the oat milk and top with the orange segments and mint leaves, if you like.

Nutrition: *per serving (with oat milk and oranges)*
kcal 363 fat 11g saturates 1g carbs 46g sugars 12g fibre 10g protein 15g salt 0g

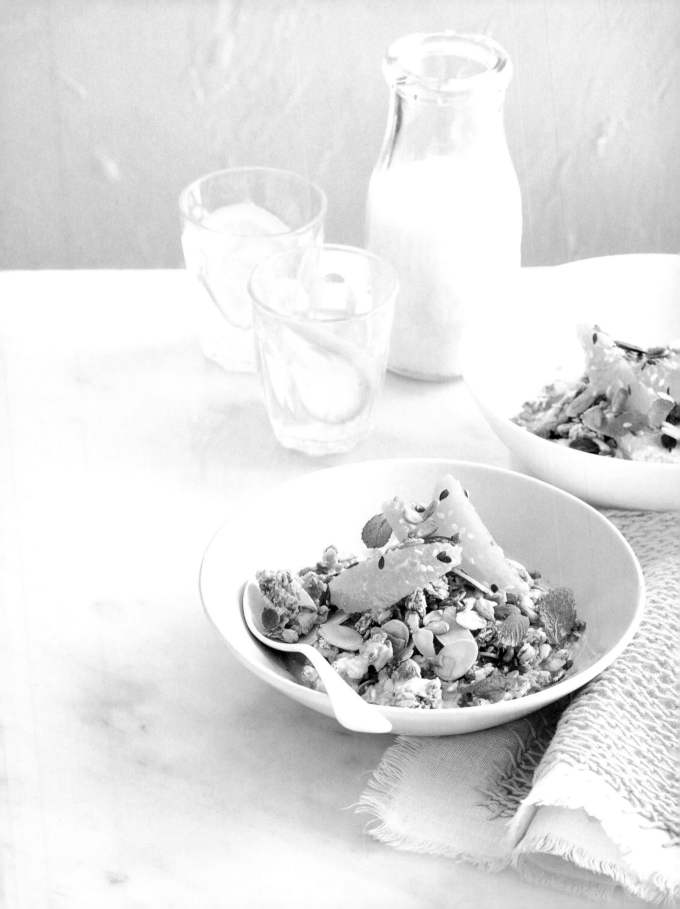

Carrot, clementine & pineapple juice

Sweet, tangy and fresh, this bright orange juice will give you a morning boost

PREP 10 mins NO COOK 1

- 1 carrot, peeled
- ½ small pineapple
- 2 clementines, peeled
- 1cm piece peeled ginger

Cut the carrot and pineapple into chunks and put in the juicer along with the clementines and ginger. Juice following the instructions for your machine. Pour into a large glass and serve.

Nutrition: *per serving*
kcal 234 fat 1g saturates 0g carbs 48g sugars 47g fibre 10g protein 3g salt 0.1g

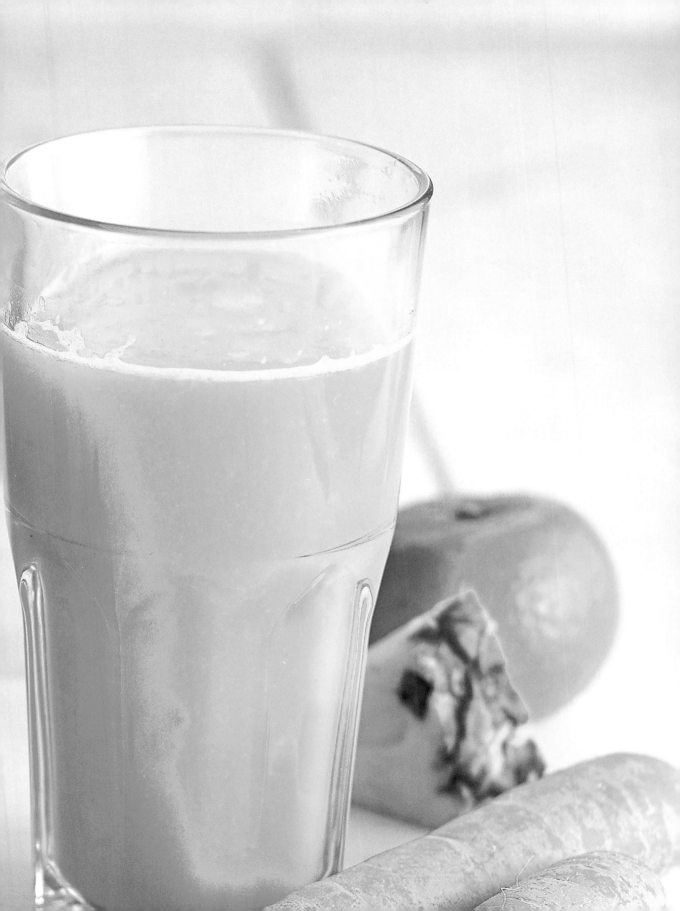

Squash steaks with chestnut & cavolo nero pilaf

This easy vegan squash recipe is deliciously spiced. Serve with a dollop of coconut yogurt.

PREP 10 mins COOK 55 mins 4

- 1 butternut squash
- 2–3 tbsp olive oil, plus extra for frying
- ½ tsp smoked paprika, plus a little extra for sprinkling
- 200g cavolo nero or curly kale, shredded
- 1 onion, chopped
- 180g chestnuts, halved
- 2 garlic cloves, finely chopped
- ½ tsp ground cumin
- ½ tsp ground cinnamon
- 250g basmati rice & wild rice
- 500ml vegetable stock
- 150g pot of coconut yogurt

1 Heat oven to 220C/200C fan/ gas 7. Cut the neck of the squash into 4 rounds (keep the rest for another time). Heat the oil in a frying pan and brown the squash for a few mins each side. Transfer to a baking tray, sprinkle with half the paprika and roast for 30 mins.

2 Meanwhile, in the same frying pan, add a little extra oil and stir-fry the cavolo nero for 2 mins, then remove with a slotted spoon and set aside. Add the onion and chestnuts to the pan, cook for a few mins, then stir in the garlic, remaining paprika and spices and cook for 1 min. Stir in the rice and stock, bring to the boil, then cover with a lid. Turn the heat down as low as it will go and cook for 25 mins, stirring occasionally.

3 Once cooked, stir through the cavolo nero and serve with the squash steaks and the coconut yogurt sprinkled with paprika.

Nutrition: *per serving*
kcal 562 fat 15g saturates 8g carbs 87g sugars 14g fibre 10g protein 14g salt 0.4g

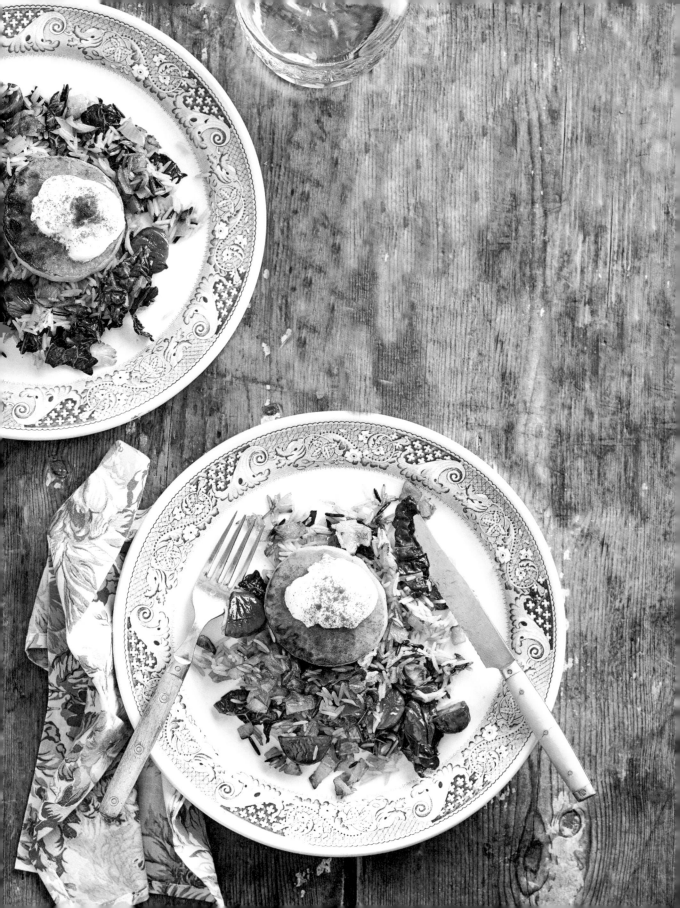

Summery stuffed squash

Just four ingredients and packed with nutrients, pick up the ingredients for this simple supper on the way home.

🕐 PREP 5 mins COOK 35 mins ◔ 2

- 1 small butternut squash
- 100g artichokes from a jar
- 100g mozzarella & sundried tomato pot
- 1 ready-to-eat grain & chickpea pouch

Heat oven to 200C/180C fan/gas 6. Halve the squash and scoop out the seeds. Put in a microwaveable bowl, cover and microwave on High for 20 mins until softening. Scoop out the flesh with a spoon, reserving the skin, and mix with the remaining ingredients. Spoon back into the skin and transfer to a baking tray. Cook for a further 10–15 mins until tender and the cheese has melted.

Nutrition: *per serving*
kcal 480 fat 18g saturates 3g carbs 55g sugars 11g fibre 14g protein 16g salt 2.3g

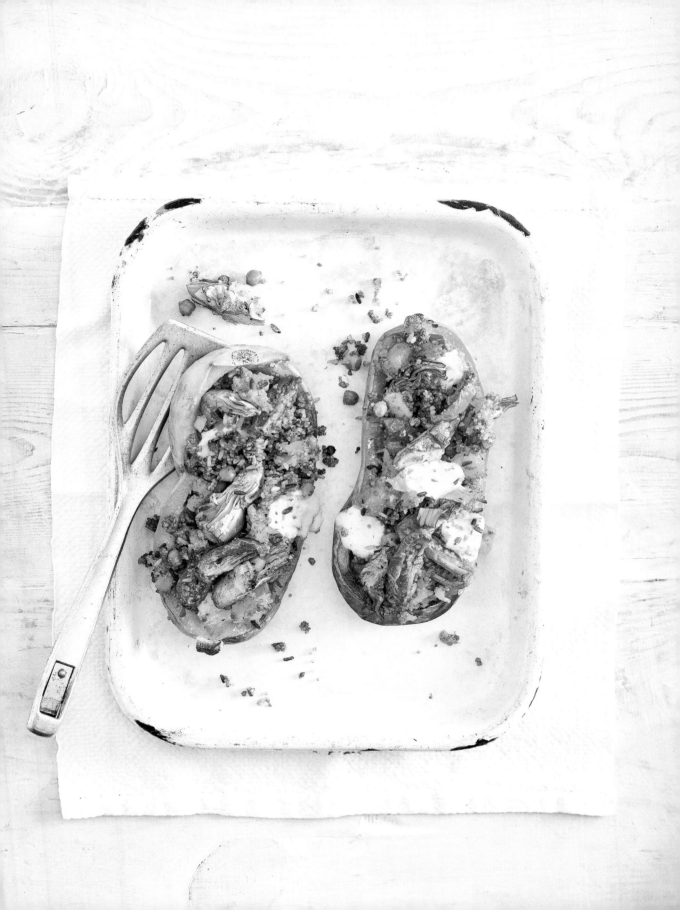

Pearl barley, parsnip & sage risotto

Wholegrain pearl barley is well worth tracking down. It'll keep for up to a year in your cupboard and has more beneficial nutrients than pearl barley.

🕐 PREP 5 mins COOK 55 mins 🕐 4

- 25g butter, plus an extra knob to stir through
- 1 onion, finely chopped
- 4 parsnips, about 500g, peeled and cut into chunks
- 1 garlic clove, crushed
- 10 sage leaves, shredded, plus extra to serve
- 400g wholegrain pearl barley, rinsed
- 1.4 litres hot vegetable stock
- 25g Parmesan (or vegetarian alternative), grated, plus extra to serve

1 Heat the butter in a large saucepan. Add the onion and a pinch of salt, and cook gently for 5 mins. Tip in the parsnips, turn up the heat and cook for 8–10 mins, stirring every so often, until the parsnips are starting to brown and caramelise.

2 Add the garlic and sage, and mix through. Tip in the barley and stir to coat well. Pour in the stock, bring to the boil, then turn down to a simmer and cook for 35–40 mins, or until nearly all the liquid has been absorbed and the pearl barley is tender but still has a bite. You may need to add a little extra boiling water.

3 Take off the heat, top with the Parmesan and a knob of butter, then leave to melt. Give the risotto a good stir, then spoon into dishes. Top with more sage, Parmesan and some black pepper.

Nutrition: *per serving*
kcal 629 fat 12g saturates 6g carbs 107g sugars 14g fibre 13g protein 15g salt 1.2g

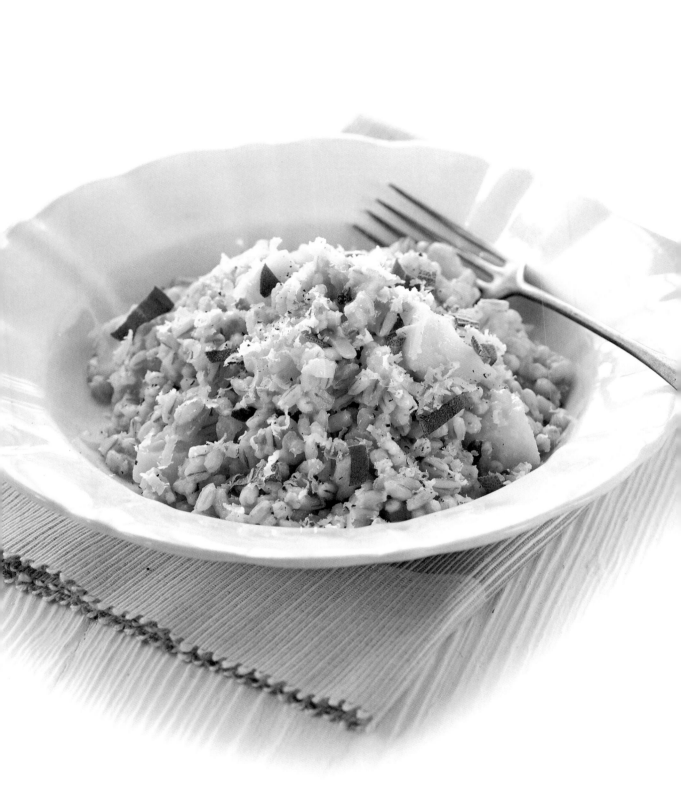

Salted maple roasted parsnips

Give your roast parsnips a sweet and salty glaze with a drizzle of maple syrup and crunchy sea salt.

PREP 5 mins COOK 40 mins 8

- 600g parsnips, peeled and quartered
- 2 tbsp vegetable oil
- 3 tbsp maple syrup
- 3 thyme sprigs, leaves picked

Heat oven to 220C/200C fan/gas 7. Put the parsnips in a large roasting tin with the oil, maple syrup, thyme leaves and some sea salt flakes. Roast for 35–40 mins until soft and sticky. Scatter over a few more sea salt flakes before serving.

Nutrition: *per serving*
kcal 97 fat 3g saturates 0g carbs 15g sugars 8g fibre 4g protein 1g salt 0g

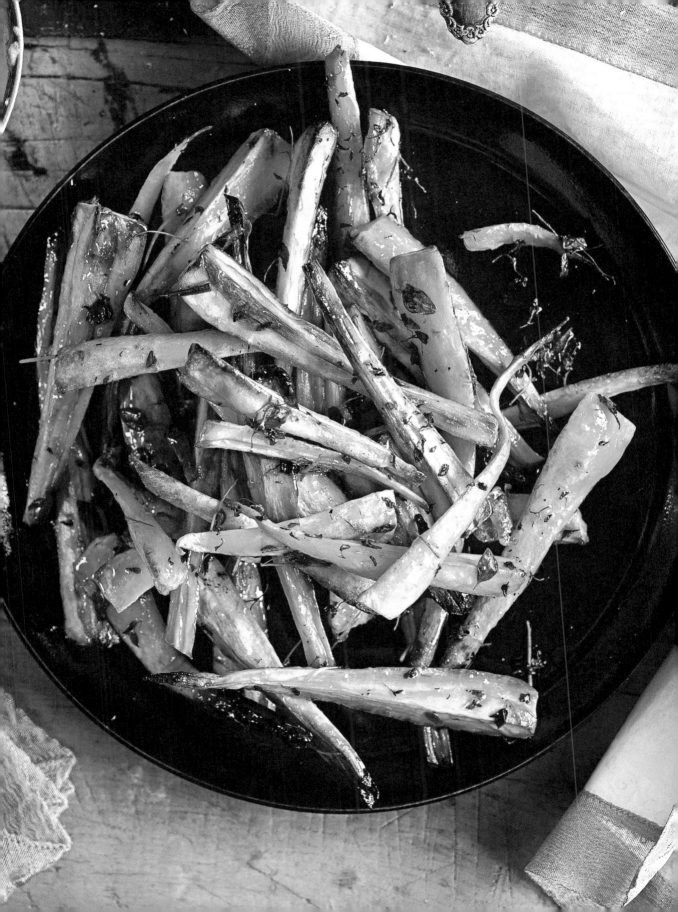

Pumpkin & bacon soup

If you can get a crown prince or onion squash, they will add a lovely sweet flavour to this soup. Butternut squash will also do the trick.

PREP 10 mins COOK 1 hr 10 mins   4

- 1 tbsp vegetable oil
- 50g butter
- 1 onion, finely chopped
- 150g maple-cured bacon, cut into small pieces
- ½ Crown Prince pumpkin or onion squash, peeled, deseeded and cut into medium chunks (you need about 500g pumpkin flesh)
- 1 litre chicken stock
- 100ml double cream
- 3 tbsp pumpkin seeds, toasted
- maple syrup, for drizzling

1 In a large, heavy-bottomed pan, heat the oil with 25g butter. Add the onion and a pinch of salt and cook on a low heat for 10 mins or until soft. Add 60g bacon and cook for a further 5 mins until the bacon releases its fat. Then increase the heat to medium, add the pumpkin and stock and season. Bring to the boil, then reduce the heat to a simmer, cover with a lid and cook for about 40 mins until the pumpkin is soft. Pour in the cream, bring to the boil again and remove from the heat. Set aside some of the liquid, then blend the remaining pumpkin until smooth and velvety, adding liquid back into the pan bit by bit as you go (add more liquid if you like it thinner). Strain through a fine sieve, check the seasoning and set aside.

2 Melt the remaining butter in a pan over a high heat and fry the rest of the bacon with black pepper for 5 mins. Divide the bacon among 4 bowls, reheat the soup and pour over. To serve, sprinkle over the pumpkin seeds and drizzle with maple syrup.

Nutrition: *per serving*
kcal 557 fat 43g saturates 20g carbs 19g sugars 12g fibre 5g protein 21g salt 2.2g

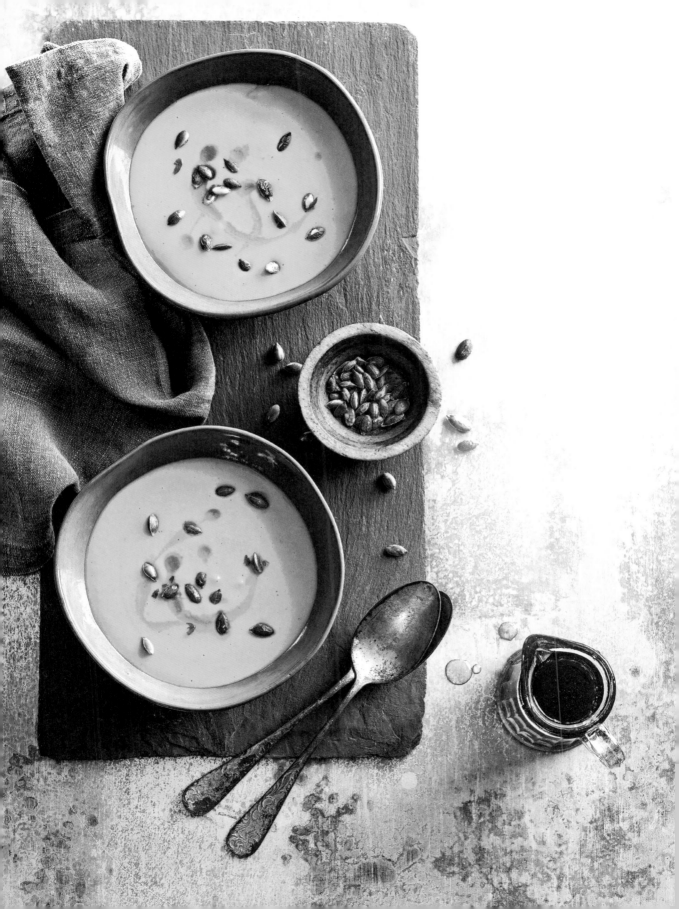

Mustard & sage chicken with celeriac mash

Replace potatoes with healthy celeriac in this hearty dinner dish.

⏱ PREP 15 mins COOK 30 mins 🥧 3

- 1 celeriac, peeled and cut into chunks
- 3 chicken breasts, skinless
- 1 tbsp English mustard powder
- 2 tsp olive oil
- 2 garlic cloves, crushed
- 8 sage leaves
- 100g crème fraîche, plus 2 tbsp for the mash
- 1 low-sodium chicken stock cube
- 2 tbsp wholegrain mustard
- 275g cooked green veg, such as thin-stemmed broccoli, peas or Savoy cabbage, to serve

1 Put the celeriac in a bowl, add a splash of water and cover with cling film. Pierce the cling film and microwave on High for 10 mins or until really tender.

2 Meanwhile, put the chicken breasts between 2 sheets of cling film and lightly bash with rolling pin until they are an even thickness. Dust with the mustard powder. Heat the oil in a large frying pan, add the chicken breasts and brown on both sides. Add the garlic and sage to the pan, stirring in the gaps between the chicken, for 30 secs– 1 min, then crumble in the stock cube.

3 Pour in 100ml hot water and add 100g crème fraîche. Stir the sauce around the chicken, then cover the pan with a lid and cook over a medium heat for 8 mins or until the chicken is cooked through. Stir through the mustard and season with plenty of black pepper.

4 While the chicken cooks, drain any liquid from the celeriac, season, add the remaining 2 tbsp crème fraîche and mash (or blitz to a purée in a food processor). Serve with the chicken and some green veg.

Nutrition: *per serving*
kcal 463 fat 26g saturates 14g carbs 10g sugars 6g fibre 14g protein 40g salt 2.3g

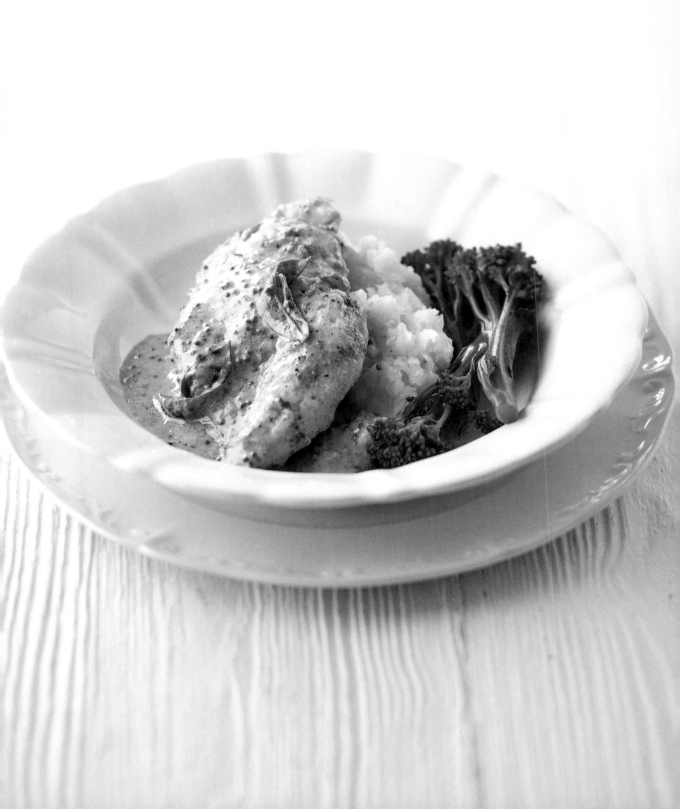

Stuffed onions

Onions get the star treatment in this dish, stuffed with lamb mince and healthy spices, they make a delicious dinner.

PREP 25 mins COOK 1 hr 25 mins 6

FOR THE ONIONS
- 4 very large onions
- 2 tbsp olive oil
- 2 tbsp pomegranate molasses

FOR THE STUFFING
- 50g Greek yogurt
- 50g fresh breadcrumbs
- 400g lamb mince (20% fat)
- 1 egg, beaten
- 1 tsp ground allspice
- ½ tsp ground cinnamon
- 1 tsp ground cumin
- 1 tsp ground coriander
- ½ small pack mint, chopped
- ½ small pack flat-leaf parsley, chopped

1 Trim the very ends of the onions. Make an incision in each, from top to root, then another 0.5cm along, so you can cut out and discard a thin wedge (like you're discarding a segment of orange). Bring a pan of water to the boil and add the onions. Boil for 10 mins, remove from the water and let cool. Heat oven to 200C/180C fan/gas 6.

2 When the onions are cool enough to handle, carefully peel and set aside their outer layers – you want about 12–16 large layers in total, which will become the outer casing for the lamb filling. You can use the smaller, leftover layers in the middle for another recipe.

3 Mix all the stuffing ingredients in a bowl and season well. Shape into 12–16 oval meatballs. Put each one on an onion layer and roll it up to create what looks like a small, peeled onion.

4 Pour half the olive oil into a large, shallow casserole dish or roasting tin, then arrange all the stuffed onions on top in a tight, single layer. Drizzle over the remaining oil and bake for 45 mins. Brush with the molasses and bake for another 15–20 mins until the casings are really soft and dark golden brown.

Nutrition: *per serving*
kcal 314 fat 19g saturates 8g carbs 18g sugars 11g fibre 4g protein 15g salt 0.3g

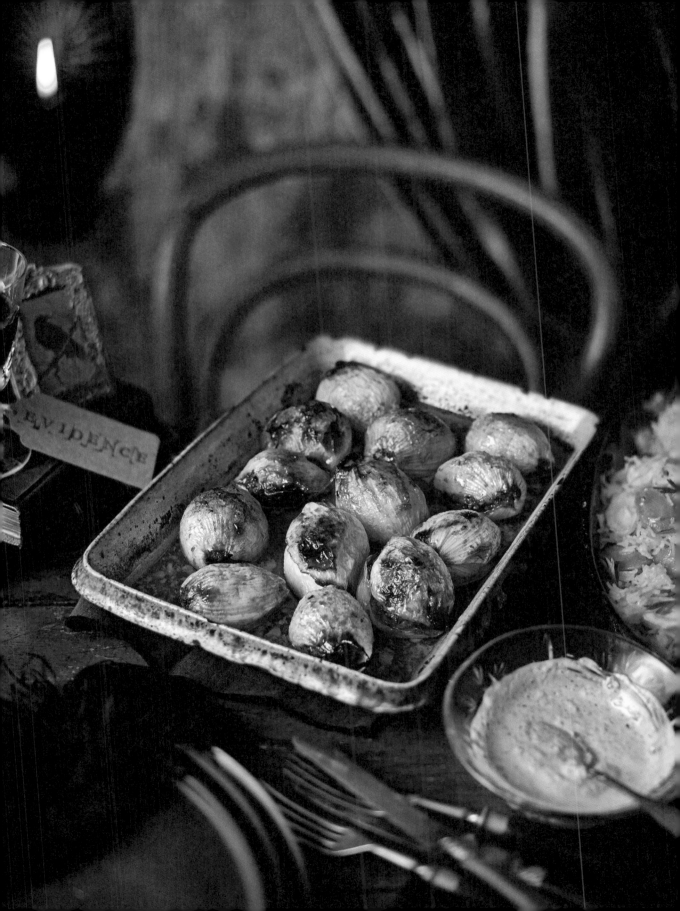

Carrot & ginger immune-boosting soup

Whizz up a healthy soup in a flash with spicy carrot and ginger.

PREP 5 mins COOK 5 mins 1

- 3 large carrots
- 1 tbsp grated ginger
- 1 tsp turmeric
- a pinch of cayenne pepper, plus extra to serve
- 20g wholemeal bread
- 1 tbsp sour cream, plus extra to serve
- 200ml vegetable stock

Peel and chop the carrots and put in a blender with the ginger, turmeric, cayenne pepper, wholemeal bread, sour cream and vegetable stock. Blitz until smooth. Heat until piping hot. Swirl through some extra sour cream, or a sprinkling of cayenne, if you like.

Nutrition: *per serving*
kcal 223 fat 7g saturates 3g carbs 30g sugars 19g fibre 10g protein 5g salt 1.1g

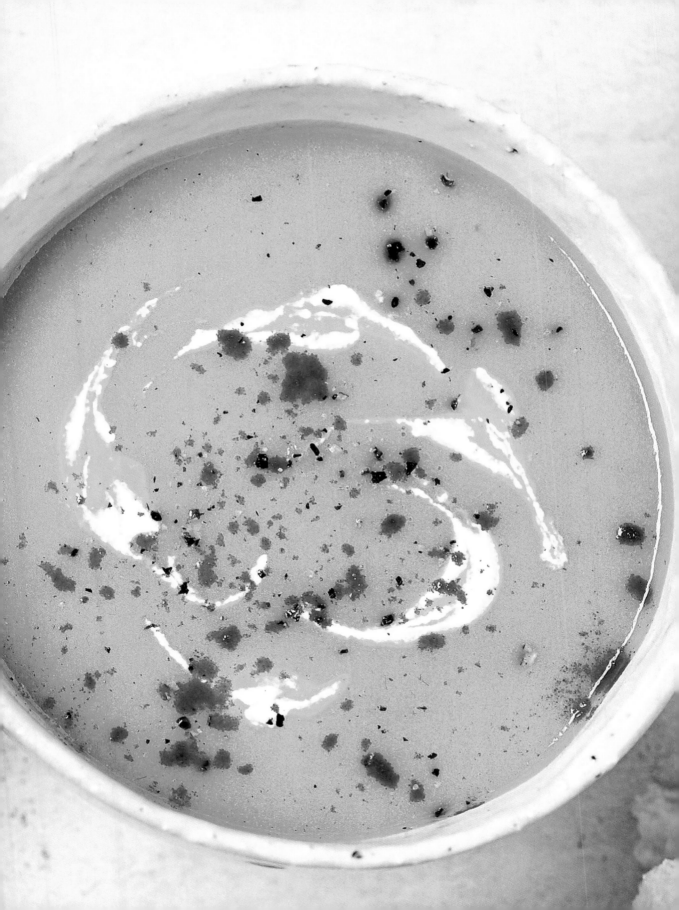

Fruity turkey tagine

This nutrient packed tagine can be made ahead and frozen for up to 3 months.

PREP 10 mins COOK 55 mins 4-6

- 1 tbsp olive oil
- 1 red onion, thickly sliced
- 3 carrots, thickly sliced on the diagonal
- 3 parsnips, thickly sliced on the diagonal
- 2 garlic cloves, crushed
- 2 tsp ras el hanout
- 500ml turkey or chicken stock
- 400g can chopped tomatoes
- 400g can chickpeas, drained and rinsed
- 140g mixture of dried apricots and prunes, roughly chopped
- 300g cooked turkey or chicken, cut into chunks
- good drizzle of clear honey
- ½ small bunch coriander, roughly chopped
- 1 tbsp flaked almonds
- couscous, to serve
- Greek yogurt, to serve

1 Heat the oil in a large saucepan, add the onion and cook gently for 8 mins or until softened. Add the carrots and parsnips, and cook for 8 mins until starting to soften and brown a little. Stir in the garlic and ras el hanout, and cook for a further 30 secs. Tip in the stock, tomatoes, chickpeas, dried fruit and 150ml water. Season, bring to a simmer and cook for 25–30 mins until the vegetables are tender.
2 Add the turkey and simmer for 5 mins to warm through. Stir in the honey, then scatter over the coriander and almonds just before serving with couscous and Greek yogurt.

Nutrition: *per serving*
kcal 343 fat 9g saturates 1g carbs 35g sugars 21g fibre 11g protein 25g salt 0.7g

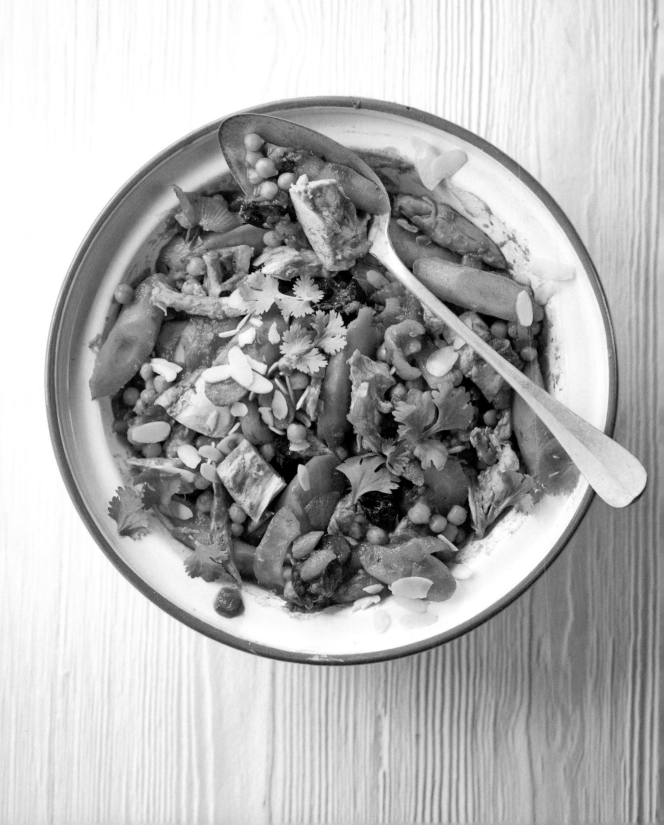

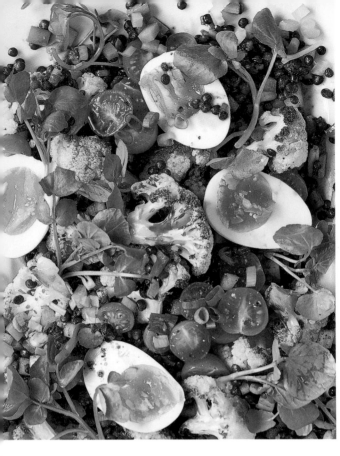
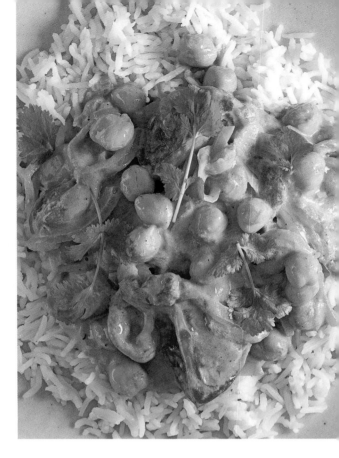
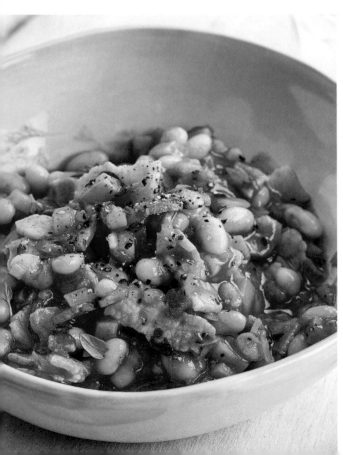
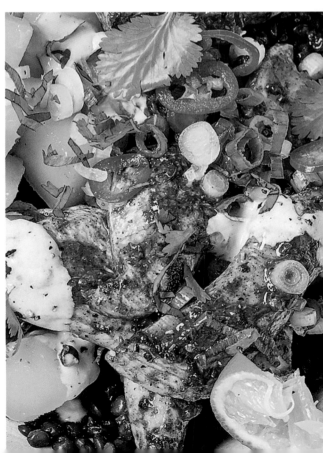

Chapter 5:

BEANS & PULSES

Low in fat, packed with protein and full of fibre, beans and pulses are loaded with superfood integrity. Lentils are a rich vegetarian source of iron as well as B vitamins and potassium for a healthy blood pressure. Try them in our Spinach, sweet potato and lentil dhal (page 198). Another source of iron as well as manganese for boosting energy levels are butter beans – we've combined them with full-flavoured chorizo in our Butter bean, chorizo & spinach baked eggs (page 218).

Black beans are often touted as the highest protein-containing bean, which makes them an ideal choice for vegetarians. We've maximized on this in our Spicy black bean tacos on page 222.

One of the most popular and versatile has to be the chickpea – high in fibre to help balance blood sugar they supply more than ten different micronutrients including the mineral copper, which promotes fabulous hair. Don't restrict them to hummus – add them to salads, casseroles and even curries – see our Tomato & chickpea curry on page 204.

It's easy to think of beans and pulses as savoury ingredients but we've got imaginative and added cannellini beans to our Carrot & Pecan muffins (page 220). Unlike most muffins ours won't leave you with sugar cravings later in the day, thanks to their high fibre content.

Spinach, sweet potato & lentil dhal

Lentils are a great store cupboard standby, if you want a speedy meal, use red lentils as they cook quickest.

PREP 10 mins COOK 35 mins 4

- 1 tbsp sesame oil
- 1 red onion, finely chopped
- 1 garlic clove, crushed
- thumb-sized piece ginger, peeled and finely chopped
- 1 red chilli, finely chopped
- 1½ tsp ground turmeric
- 1½ tsp ground cumin
- 2 sweet potatoes (about 400g), cut into even chunks
- 250g red split lentils
- 600ml vegetable stock
- 80g bag of spinach
- 4 spring onions, sliced on the diagonal, to serve
- ½ small pack of Thai basil, leaves torn, to serve

1 Heat the oil in a wide-based pan with a tight-fitting lid. Add the onion and cook over a low heat for 10 mins, stirring occasionally, until softened. Add the garlic, ginger and chilli, cook for 1 min, then add the spices and cook for 1 min more.

2 Turn up the heat to medium, add the sweet potato and stir everything together so the potato is coated in the spice mixture. Tip in the lentils, stock and some seasoning. Bring the liquid to the boil, then reduce the heat, cover and cook for 20 mins until the lentils are tender and the potato is just holding its shape

3 Taste and adjust the seasoning, then gently stir in the spinach. Once wilted, top with the spring onions and basil to serve. Or allow to cool completely, then divide among airtight containers and store in the fridge for a healthy lunchbox.

Nutrition: *per serving*
kcal 397 fat 5g saturates 1g carbs 65g sugars 19g fibre 11g protein 18g salt 0.6g

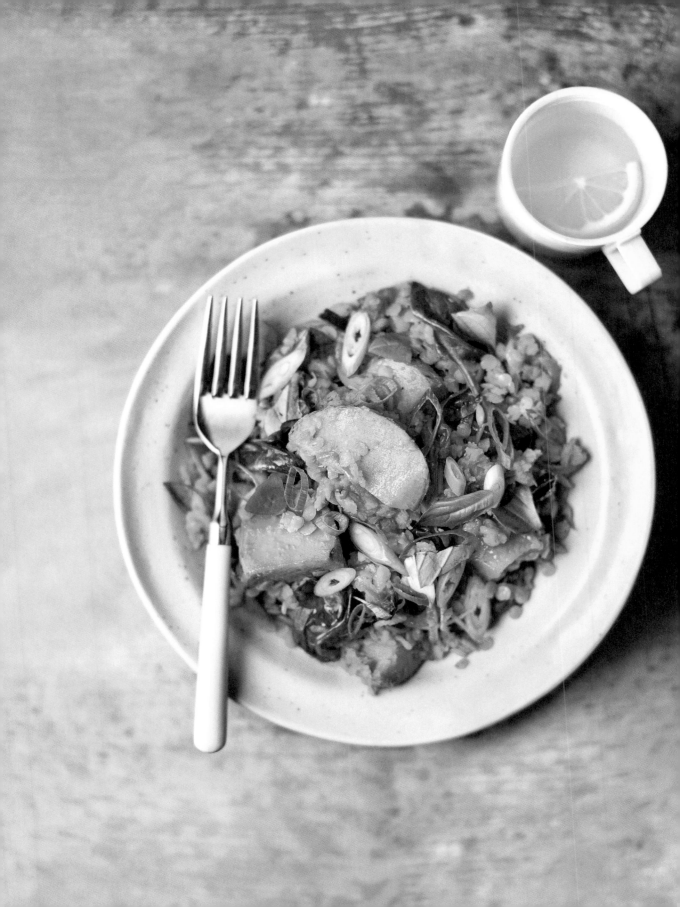

Egg & puy lentil salad with tamari & watercress

This is the ultimate healthy recipe to ease the symptoms of menopause, packed with calcium, folate and iron.

PREP 10 mins plus soaking COOK 35 mins | 2

- 75g dried Puy lentils
- 175g cauliflower florets, broken into smaller pieces
- 1 tbsp rapeseed oil, plus a drizzle
- 1 large carrot, chopped into small pieces
- 2 celery sticks, chopped into small pieces
- 2 garlic cloves
- 3 eggs
- 1 tbsp tamari or soy sauce
- 10 cherry tomatoes, halved
- 4 spring onions, finely sliced
- 2 generous handfuls watercress, large stems removed

1 Soak the lentils in cold water for 8 hrs, or overnight.

2 When ready to eat, drain the lentils and heat oven to 220C/200C fan/gas 7. Toss the cauliflower with a drizzle of the oil, then roast for 20 mins on a parchment-lined baking tray until tender and tinged with gold round the edges.

3 Meanwhile, put the drained lentils in a pan with the carrot and celery. Pour in water to cover, put on a lid and boil for 20 mins until the lentils are tender. Check before they are ready in case they are boiling dry and, if necessary, top up with a little more water.

4 While they are cooking, finely grate the garlic and set aside in a large bowl. Boil the eggs for 6 mins, this will give you eggs with a soft yolk. When they are ready, plunge into cold water, then shell.

5 Mix the tamari and oil into the garlic to make a dressing. Check the lentils and drain, if necessary, then toss in the bowl with the dressing, tomatoes, spring onions and watercress. Pile onto plates and top with the eggs, adding any remaining dressing from the bowl over the top.

Nutrition: *per serving*
kcal 411 fat 18g saturates 3g carbs 30g sugars 11g fibre 12g protein 26g salt 1.6g

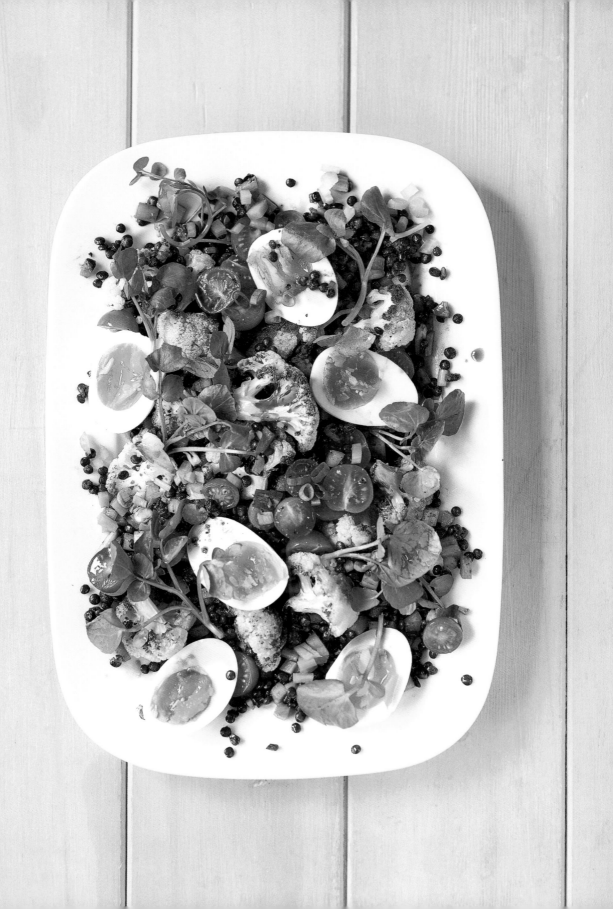

Halloumi with lemony lentils, chickpeas & beets

A great storecupboard salad, topped with golden brown halloumi and quick, homemade pickled red onion.

PREP 15 mins COOK 30 mins 4

- 200g Puy lentils
- 2 lemons
- 1 red onion, finely sliced
- 3 tbsp extra virgin olive oil
- 3 tbsp capers, very roughly chopped
- 400g can chickpeas, drained and rinsed
- 250g cooked beetroot, cut into matchsticks
- ½ small pack parsley, roughly chopped
- 250g pack halloumi, cut into 8 slices

1 Cook the lentils in a pan of boiling water for 20–25 mins or until just done. Meanwhile, squeeze the juice from one lemon into a bowl. Add the onion and scrunch together with a pinch of salt to pickle slightly. Set aside.
2 Finely zest the remaining lemon and set aside for the halloumi. Squeeze the juice into a jam jar or jug. Add the oil with a pinch of seasoning and the capers – shake well and set aside. When the lentils are ready, drain and tip into a large serving bowl with the chickpeas. Toss with the dressing straight away, then toss through the beets, parsley, pickled onions and their juice.
3 Heat a frying pan over a medium heat and fry the halloumi for 1–2 mins each side or until golden brown. Toss with the lemon zest, then place on top of your salad to serve.

Nutrition: *per serving*
kcal 559 fat 26g saturates 12g carbs 42g sugars 9g fibre 12g protein 33g salt 2.5g

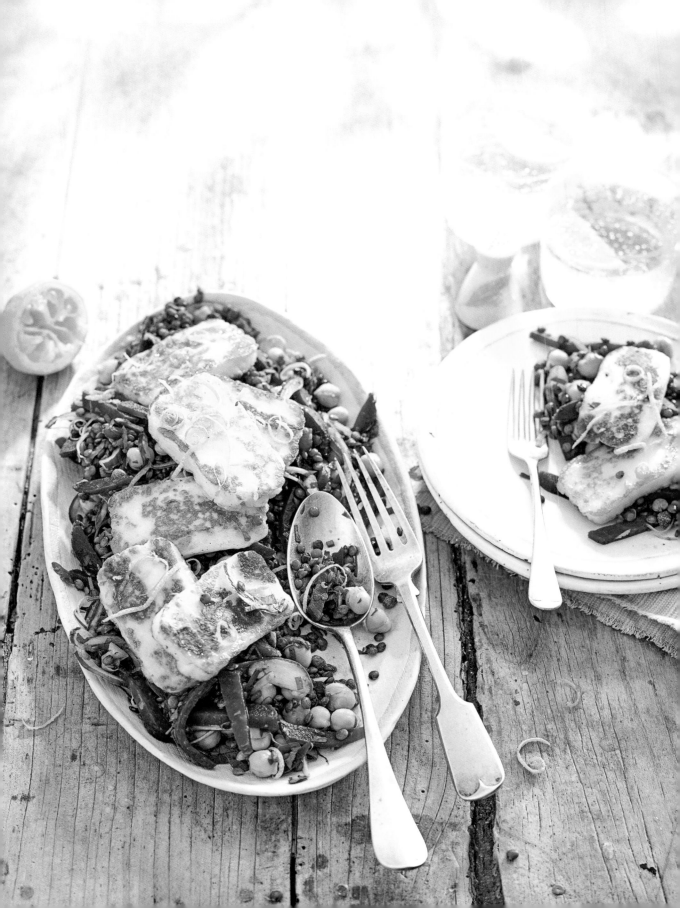

Tomato & chickpea curry

Want to use up the cans cluttering up your cupboards? This satisfying veggie chickpea curry is made in three easy steps and counts as 3 of your 5-a-day

PREP 10 mins COOK 45 mins 4

- 1 tbsp olive oil
- 2 onions, finely sliced
- 2 garlic cloves, crushed
- 1 tsp garam masala
- 1 tsp turmeric
- 1 tsp ground coriander
- 400g can plum tomatoes
- 400ml can coconut milk
- 400g can chickpeas, drained and rinsed
- 2 large tomatoes, quartered
- ½ small pack coriander, roughly chopped
- cooked basmati rice, to serve

1 Heat the oil in a large pan and add the onions. Cook until softened, about 10 mins. Add the garlic and spices, and stir to combine. Cook for 1–2 mins, then pour in the canned tomatoes, break up with a wooden spoon and simmer for 10 mins.

2 Pour in the coconut milk and season. Bring to the boil and simmer for a further 10–15 mins until the sauce has thickened.

3 Tip in the chickpeas and the tomatoes, and warm through. Scatter over the coriander and serve with fluffy rice.

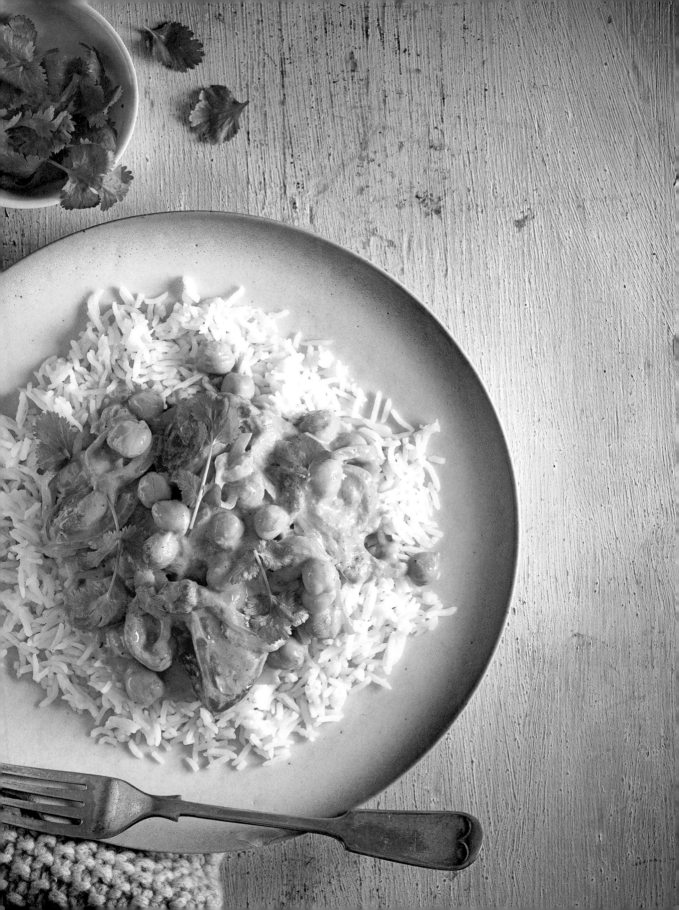

Jerk chicken & mango bowl

A fruity chicken salad with lentils and spice to make lunchtimes worth taking a break for.

PREP 15 mins COOK 15 mins 2

- 2 chicken breasts, cut into strips
- 2 tbsp jerk paste
- 1 tbsp olive oil
- 250g ready-to-eat Puy lentils
- 4 spring onions, finely sliced
- I red chilli, sliced
- ½ small bunch coriander, leaves only
- 1 mango, cubed
- 1 lime, cut into wedges
- 8 tbsp natural yogurt
- 4 tbsp mango chutney

1 Heat oven to 200C/180C fan/ gas 6. Put the chicken in a roasting tin and rub with the jerk paste, olive oil and a little seasoning. Bake for 15 mins until it is cooked, then leave to cool.

2 Build each bowl by putting half the lentils, chicken, spring onions, chilli, coriander and mango in each, with lime wedges at the side. Put yogurt in a separate pot with the mango chutney swirled through. Coat in the yogurt dressing just before eating.

Nutrition: *per serving*
kcal 660 fat 18g saturates 5g carbs 66g sugars 39g fibre 11g protein 54g salt 3.3g

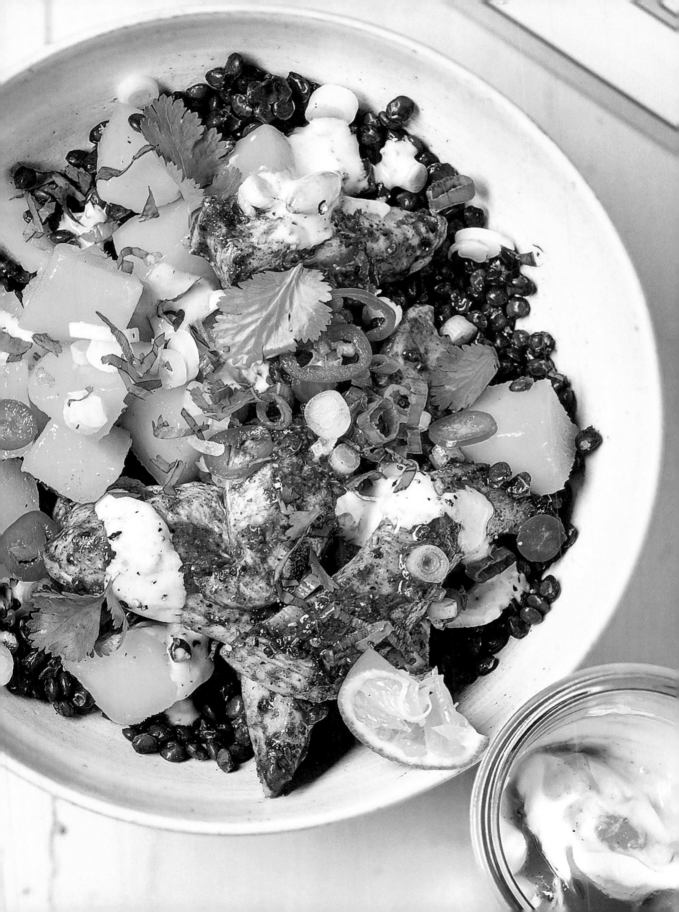

Pesto crusted cod with puy lentils

You can replace the cod in this recipe with any fish you fancy, salmon or mackerel would give you a good omega-3 boost.

PREP 15 mins COOK 10 mins 2

- large pack basil, leaves only
- 4 garlic cloves, 2 whole, 2 crushed
- 25g pine nuts
- 1 lemon
- 50ml olive oil
- 2 cod fillets
- 2 red chillies, finely chopped
- 2 large tomatoes, roughly chopped
- 250g ready-to-eat Puy lentils

1 First, make the pesto. In a food processor, pulse the basil, whole garlic cloves, pine nuts, the juice of ½ the lemon and some seasoning, gradually adding most of the oil. Taste and adjust the seasoning.

2 Heat oven to 180C/160C fan/ gas 4 and line a roasting tin with foil. Season the cod on both sides and coat each fillet in the pesto. Cook for 8–10 mins until a crust has formed and the cod is cooked through.

3 Meanwhile, heat the remaining oil in a small saucepan. Add the crushed garlic and the chillies, and cook for a couple of mins to release the flavour. Add the tomatoes and cook for 1 min more. Tip in the lentils, squeeze over the other ½ of the lemon, then season. Cook until piping hot and serve with the pesto cod.

Nutrition: *per serving*
kcal 672 fat 37g saturates 5g carbs 34g sugars 7g fibre 11g protein 45g salt 1.6g

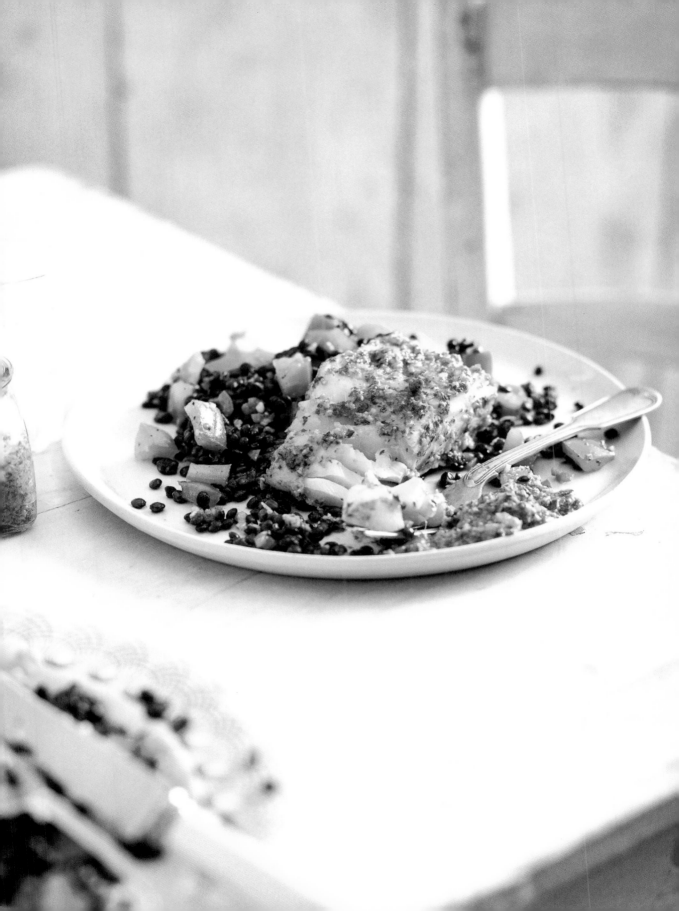

Lentil ragu with courgetti

Struggle to get your five-a-day? This superhealthy ragu will get you four steps closer and can be frozen for extra convenience.

PREP 15 mins COOK 45 mins 4

- 2 tbsp extra virgin rapeseed oil, plus 1 tsp
- 3 celery sticks, chopped
- 2 carrots, chopped
- 4 garlic cloves, chopped
- 2 onions, finely chopped
- 140g button mushrooms, quartered
- 500g pack dried red lentils
- 500g carton passata
- 1 litre reduced-salt vegetable bouillon (we used Marigold)
- 1 tsp dried oregano
- 2 tbsp balsamic vinegar
- 1–2 large courgettes, cut into noodles with a spiraliser, julienne peeler or knife

1 Heat the 2 tbsp oil in a large sauté pan. Add the celery, carrots, garlic and onions, and fry for 4–5 mins over a high heat to soften and start to colour. Add the mushrooms and fry for 2 mins more.

2 Stir in the lentils, passata, bouillon, oregano and balsamic vinegar. Cover the pan and leave to simmer for 30 mins until the lentils are tender and pulpy. Check occasionally and stir to make sure the mixture isn't sticking to the bottom of the pan; if it does, add a drop of water.

3 To serve, heat the remaining oil in a separate frying pan, add the courgette and stir-fry briefly to soften and warm through. Serve half the ragu with the courgetti and chill the rest to eat on another day. Can be frozen for up to 3 months.

Nutrition: *per serving*
kcal 578 fat 7g saturates 1g carbs 87g sugars 19g fibre 14g protein 35g salt 0.2g

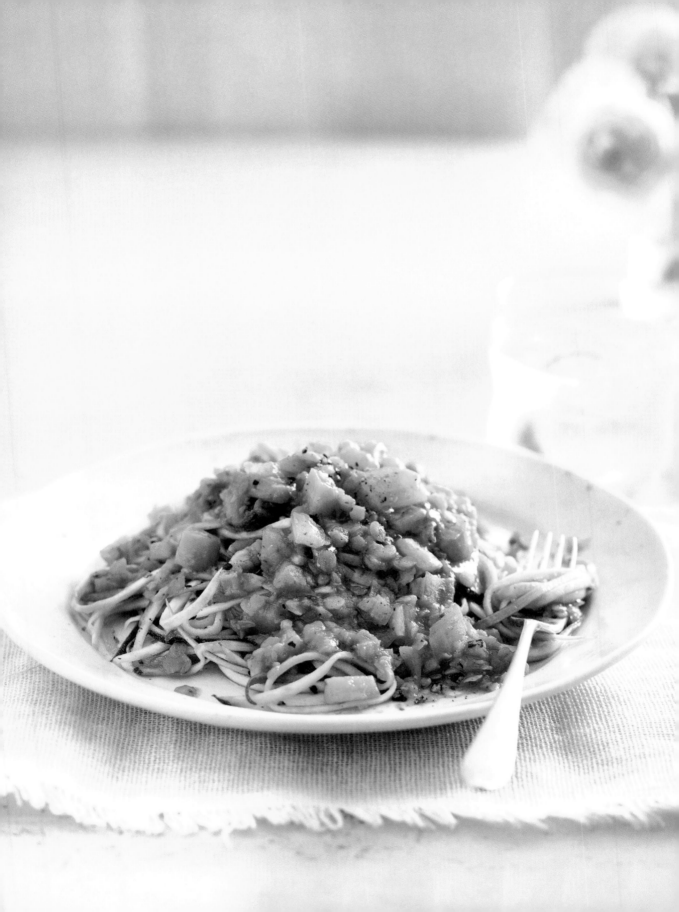

Creamy black dhal with crispy onions

This super-satisfying, slow cooked curry is packed with iron and fibre. Serve with a choice of tasty garnishes to turn your simple supper into a warming feast.

PREP 30 mins plus soaking 2 hours 30 mins | 4

- 250g black urid beans (also called urid dal, urad dal, black lentils or black gram beans – available from large supermarkets) – yellow split peas also work well
- 100g butter or ghee
- 2 large white onions, halved and thinly sliced
- 3 garlic cloves, crushed
- thumb-sized piece ginger, peeled and finely chopped
- 2 tsp ground cumin
- 2 tsp ground coriander
- 1 tsp ground turmeric
- 1 tsp paprika
- ¼ tsp chilli powder (optional)
- small bunch coriander, stalks finely chopped, leaves reserved to serve
- 400g carton passata or chopped tomatoes
- 1 fat red chilli, pierced a few times with the tip of a sharp knife
- 50ml double cream
- cooked rice, naan bread or baked sweet potatoes and crispy onions, to serve

1 Soak the beans in cold water for 4 hrs (or overnight, if you like).

2 Melt the butter or ghee in a large pan, then add the onions, garlic and ginger, and cook slowly for 10–15 mins until the onions are starting to caramelise. Stir in the spices, coriander stalks and 100ml water. Add the passata and whole red chilli. Drain the beans and add these too, then top up with 400ml water. Cover and cook for 2 hrs over a very low heat on the hob. Stir every 30 mins or so, and top up with a little more water if the dhal looks dry.

3 Once cooked, the dhal should be very thick and the beans tender. Stir in the cream, check the seasoning and serve in bowls with naan bread, rice or in a jacket potato, with coriander and crispy onions. To freeze the dhal, cool completely, then divide into containers or sandwich bags. Freeze for up to 2 months, defrost and heat thoroughly before eating.

Nutrition: *per serving*
kcal 527 fat 34g saturates 21g carbs 35g sugars 9g fibre 6g protein 19g salt 0.1g

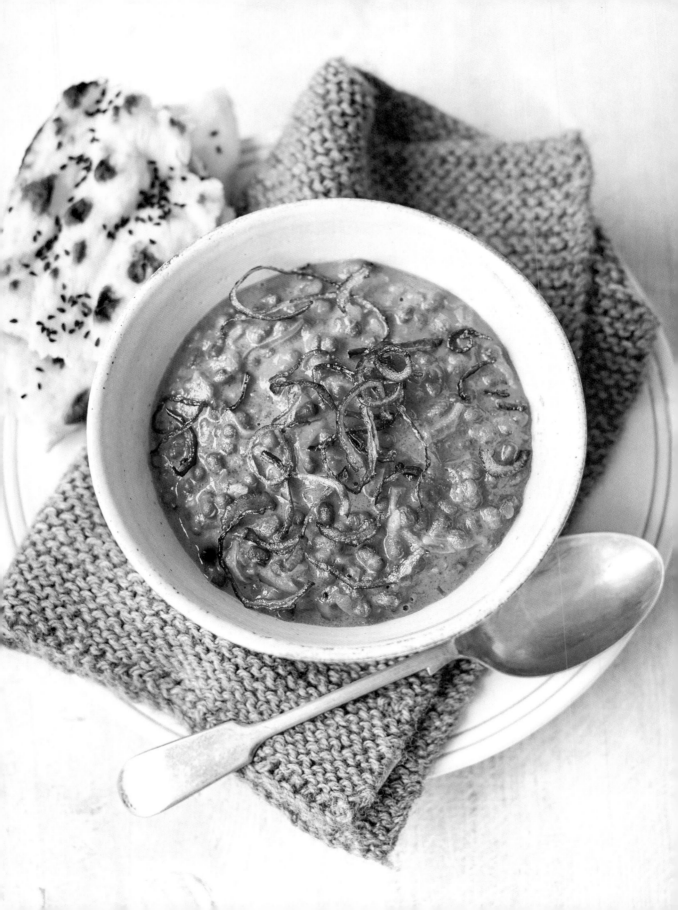

Moroccan vegetable stew

This warming one-pot stew is packed with nourishing ingredients like fibre-full chickpeas and iron-rich lentils.

PREP 30 mins COOK 35 mins 4

- 1 tbsp extra virgin rapeseed oil
- 1 medium onion, finely sliced
- 2 thin leeks, trimmed and cut into thick slices
- 2 large garlic cloves, finely sliced
- 2 tsp ground coriander
- 2 tsp ground cumin
- ½ tsp chilli flakes
- ¼ tsp ground cinnamon
- 400g can chopped tomatoes
- 1 red pepper, deseeded and cut into chunks
- 1 yellow pepper, deseeded and cut into chunks
- 400g can chickpeas drained and rinsed
- 100g dried split red lentils
- 375g sweet potatoes, peeled and cut into chunks
- juice 1 large orange plus peel, thickly sliced with a vegetable peeler
- 50g mixed nuts, such as brazils, hazelnuts, pecans and walnuts, toasted and roughly chopped
- ½ small pack coriander, roughly chopped, to serve
- full-fat natural bio-yogurt, to serve (optional)

1 Heat the oil in a large flameproof casserole or saucepan and gently fry the onion and leeks for 10–15 mins until well softened, stirring occasionally. Add the garlic and cook for 2 mins more.

2 Stir in the ground coriander, cumin, chilli and cinnamon. Cook for 2 mins, stirring occasionally. Season with plenty of ground black pepper. Add the chopped tomatoes, peppers, chickpeas, lentils, sweet potatoes, orange peel and juice, half the nuts and 400ml water and bring to a simmer. Cook for 15 mins, adding a splash of water if the stew looks too dry, and stir occasionally until the potatoes are softened but not breaking apart.

3 Remove the pan from the heat and ladle the stew into bowls. Scatter with coriander and the remaining nuts and top with yogurt, if using.

Nutrition: *per serving (excluding yogurt)*
kcal 482 fat 14g saturates 2g carbs 63g sugars 26g fibre 15g protein 18g salt 0.6g

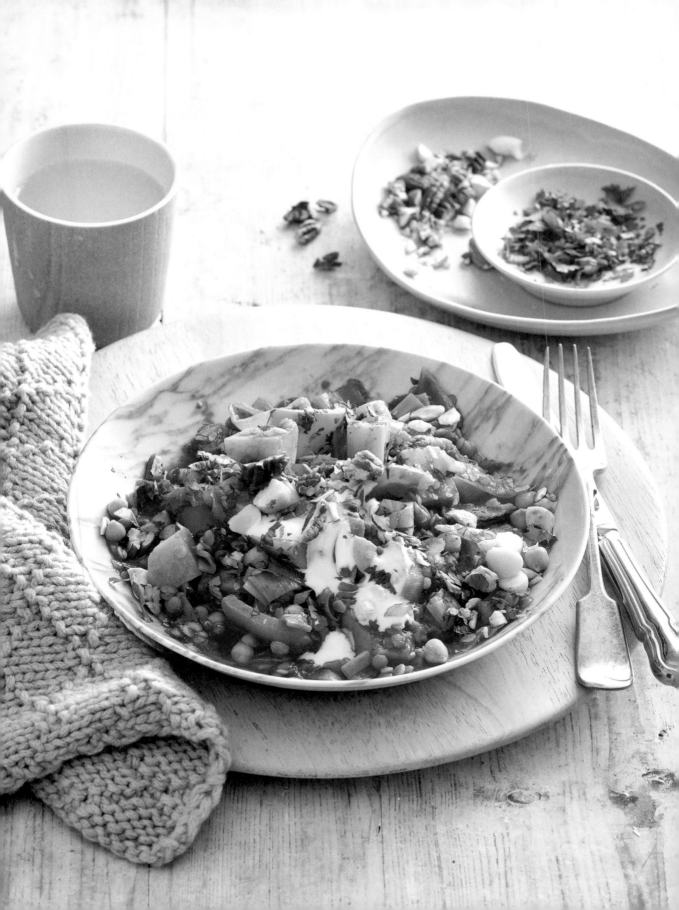

Lentil kofta with orzo & feta

Middle-Eastern inspired vegetarian 'meatballs' pair perfectly with orzo pasta and creamy feta cheese – a deliciously different everyday dinner.

PREP 25 mins plus chilling COOK 30 mins 4

- 2 x 400g cans cooked green lentils, drained
- 1 medium egg
- 100g oats
- 1 tbsp ras el hanout
- small bunch parsley, chopped
- zest 1 lemon
- 2 tbsp olive or extra virgin rapeseed oil
- 4 garlic cloves, crushed
- 2 x 400g cans chopped tomatoes
- pinch of sugar
- 300g orzo pasta
- 100g feta, crumbled

1 Put the lentils, egg, oats, ras el hanout, half the parsley and the lemon zest in a food processer. Add some seasoning and blitz until finely chopped. Remove the blade, shape the mixture into balls the size of cherry tomatoes, then chill for 20 mins. Heat oven to 200C/180C fan/gas 6.

2 Meanwhile, heat 1 tbsp of the oil in a pan. Add the garlic, sizzle for 30 secs, then add the tomatoes, sugar and some seasoning. Bubble the sauce for 20–25 mins until rich and thickened. While the sauce cooks, line a baking tray with foil and arrange the kofta on top. Drizzle over the remaining oil, and bake for 20 mins, rolling around in the tray halfway through cooking. Once cooked, add the kofta to the tomato sauce, gently coating each one.

3 Cook the orzo following pack instructions, then drain and divide amongst 4 plates. Top with the sauce and kofta, crumble over the feta and sprinkle with the remaining parsley.

Nutrition: *per serving*
kcal 598 fat 16g saturates 5g carbs 82g sugars 8g fibre 11g protein 26g salt 1.3g

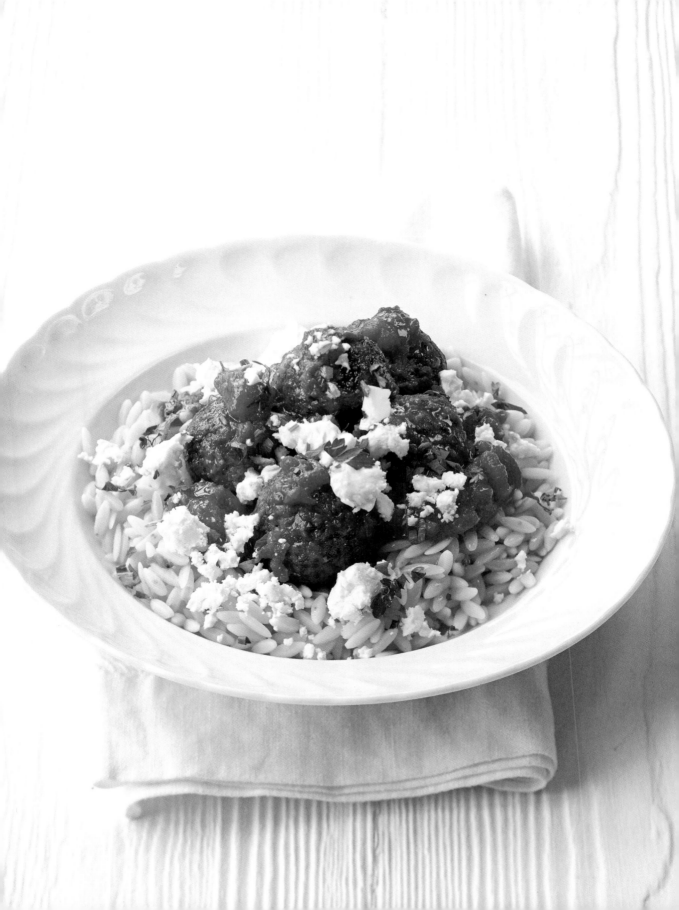

Butter bean, chorizo & spinach baked eggs

Tinned beans are a great way to get more beans and pulses in your diet. You can swap the butter beans in this dish for any beans you like.

⏱ PREP 5 mins COOK 15 mins 🥧 2

- ½ tbsp olive oil
- 1 red onion, sliced
- 1 garlic clove, chopped
- 1 tsp chilli flakes
- 100g chorizo, sliced into thin rounds
- 400g can butter beans, drained
- 100g spinach
- 4 medium eggs
- small handful coriander (optional)

1 Heat oven to 220C/200C fan/gas 7. Heat the oil in a medium frying pan (ovenproof if you have one) over a medium heat. Add the onion and cook for 3 mins until starting to soften.

2 Add the garlic, chilli flakes and chorizo, and fry for another 2 mins before adding the butter beans and a generous pinch of salt. Stir to combine, then cook for 2 mins more. Add the spinach and a splash of water and stir until wilted. Remove from the heat.

3 If your pan isn't ovenproof, tip the mixture into a medium casserole dish. Make 4 dips in the mixture with the back of a tablespoon and crack the eggs into each hole. Sprinkle with salt and freshly ground pepper (and extra chilli, if you like), then bake for 5–6 mins until the egg whites are set and the yolk is still runny. Serve with a scattering of chopped coriander, if you like.

Nutrition: *per serving*
kcal 504 fat 29g saturates 9g carbs 22g sugars 6g fibre 9g protein 34g salt 2.3g

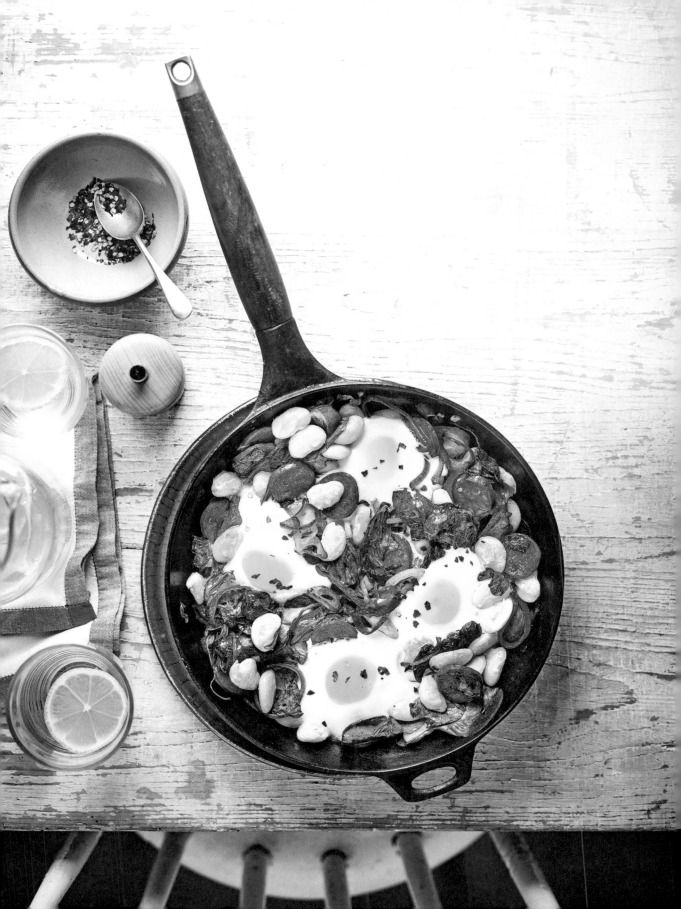

Carrot & pecan muffins

Based on the flavours of carrot cake, these have a surprise ingredient – cannellini beans!
They add a lovely texture and help provide 1 of your 5 a day.

PREP 10 mins COOK 20 mins | 12

- 2 x 400g cans cannellini beans in water, drained
- 2 tsp ground cinnamon
- 100g porridge oats
- 4 large eggs
- 2 tbsp extra virgin rapeseed oil
- 4 tbsp maple syrup
- 2 tsp vanilla extract
- zest 1 large orange
- 170g carrots, coarsely grated
- 100g raisins
- 80g pecan halves, 12 reserved, the rest roughly chopped
- 2 tsp baking powder

1 Heat oven to 180C/160C fan/gas 4 and line a 12-hole muffin tin with paper cases. Tip the beans into a bowl and add the cinnamon, oats, eggs, oil, maple syrup, vanilla extract and orange zest. Blitz with a hand blender until really smooth – the beans and oats should be ground down as much as possible.
2 Stir in the carrot, raisins, chopped pecans and baking powder, and mix well. Spoon into the muffin cases – use a large ice cream scoop if you have one, to get nice even muffins.
3 Top each muffin with a reserved pecan and bake for 20 mins until set and light brown. Cool on a wire rack. Will keep in the fridge for a few days, or freeze for 6 weeks; thaw at room temperature.

Nutrition: *per muffin*
kcal 209 fat 9g saturates 1g carbs 22g sugars 11g fibre 5g protein 7g salt 0.3g

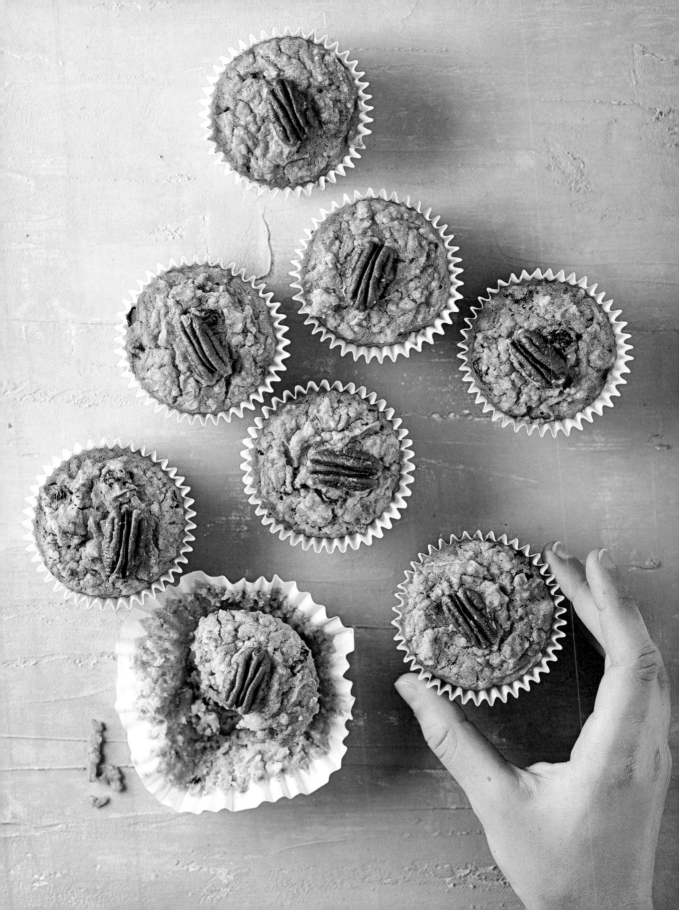

Spicy black bean tacos

These vegetarian bean tacos, lightly spiced with cumin and smoked paprika, are topped with fresh guacamole and a pomegranate salsa.

PREP 15 mins COOK 10 mins | 4

- 1 tbsp vegetable oil
- 3 garlic cloves, chopped
- 3 x 400g cans black beans, drained and rinsed
- 3 tbsp cider vinegar
- 1½ tbsp honey
- 1½ tbsp smoked paprika
- 1½ tbsp ground cumin

FOR THE GUACAMOLE
- 1 small garlic clove
- 2 tbsp roughly chopped coriander
- 1 green chilli, sliced
- 2 avocados, peeled, halved and stoned
- juice 1 lime

FOR THE SALSA
- 110g pack pomegranate seeds
- 1 green chilli, finely diced
- 1 small white onion, finely diced
- small handful fresh coriander, chopped

TO SERVE
- 8–12 corn or flour tortillas
- chipotle or other hot sauce
- soured cream or coconut yogurt

1 In a large frying pan, heat the oil and add the garlic. Fry until golden, then add the beans. Pour in the cider vinegar, honey and spices along with 1 tsp or more of salt, to taste. Cook until warmed through, crushing gently with the back of your wooden spoon, then set aside.
2 The best way to make the guacamole is with a large stone pestle and mortar, but you can use a medium bowl and a flat-ended rolling pin instead. Crush the garlic, coriander and chilli into a rough paste. Scoop in the avocado with a little salt and crush roughly – you want it chunky, not smooth. Squeeze in the lime juice and set aside.
3 Mix the salsa ingredients in a small bowl. Heat a griddle pan or steamer and quickly griddle the tortillas or steam a stack of them to warm up. Reheat the bean mixture.
4 To serve, put 1–2 heaped tbsp of beans on a tortilla. Top with a big spoonful of guacamole and some salsa, hot sauce and a dollop of soured cream or yogurt.

Nutrition: *per serving*
kcal 640 fat 24g saturates 5g carbs 74g sugars 12g fibre 18g protein 21g salt 2.7g

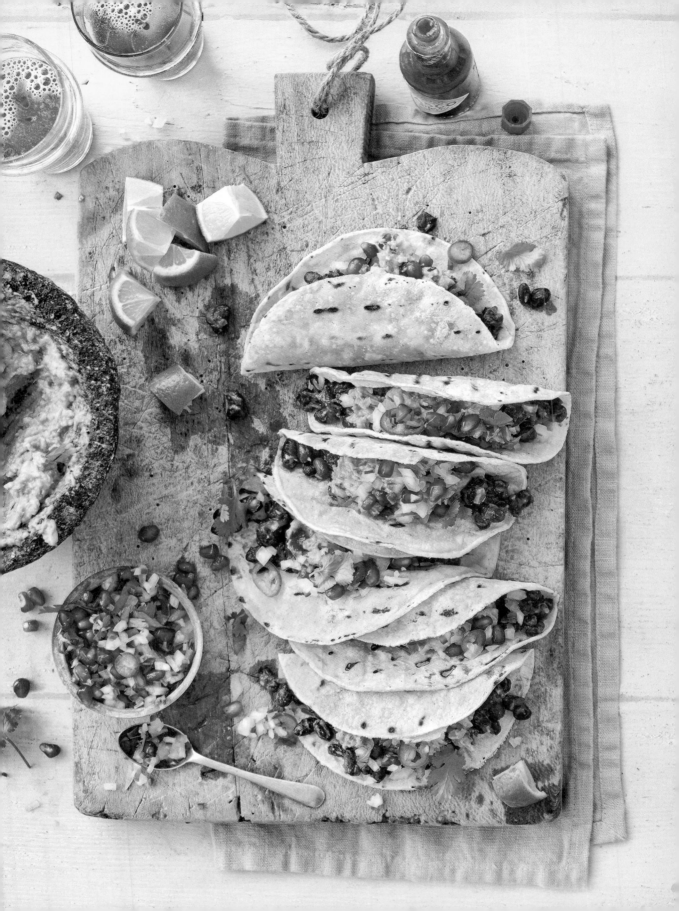

Kidney bean curry

A rescue recipe for when there's nothing in the fridge, or when you fancy something cheap, delicious and filling.

PREP 5 mins COOK 30 mins | 2

- 1 tbsp vegetable oil
- 1 onion, finely chopped
- 2 garlic cloves, finely chopped
- thumb-sized piece of ginger, peeled and finely chopped
- 1 small pack coriander, stalks finely chopped, leaves roughly shredded
- 1 tsp ground cumin
- 1 tsp ground paprika
- 2 tsp garam masala
- 400g can chopped tomatoes
- 400g can kidney beans, in water
- cooked basmati rice, to serve

1 Heat the oil in a large frying pan over a low-medium heat. Add the onion and a pinch of salt and cook slowly, stirring occasionally, until softened and just starting to colour. Add the garlic, ginger and coriander stalks and cook for a further 2 mins, until fragrant.

2 Add the spices to the pan and cook for another 1 min, by which point everything should smell aromatic. Tip in the chopped tomatoes and kidney beans in their water, then bring to the boil.

3 Turn down the heat and simmer for 15 mins until the curry is nice and thick. Season to taste, then serve with the basmati rice and the coriander leaves.

Nutrition: *per serving*
kcal 282 fat 8g saturates 1g carbs 33g sugars 13g fibre 14g protein 13g salt 0.1g

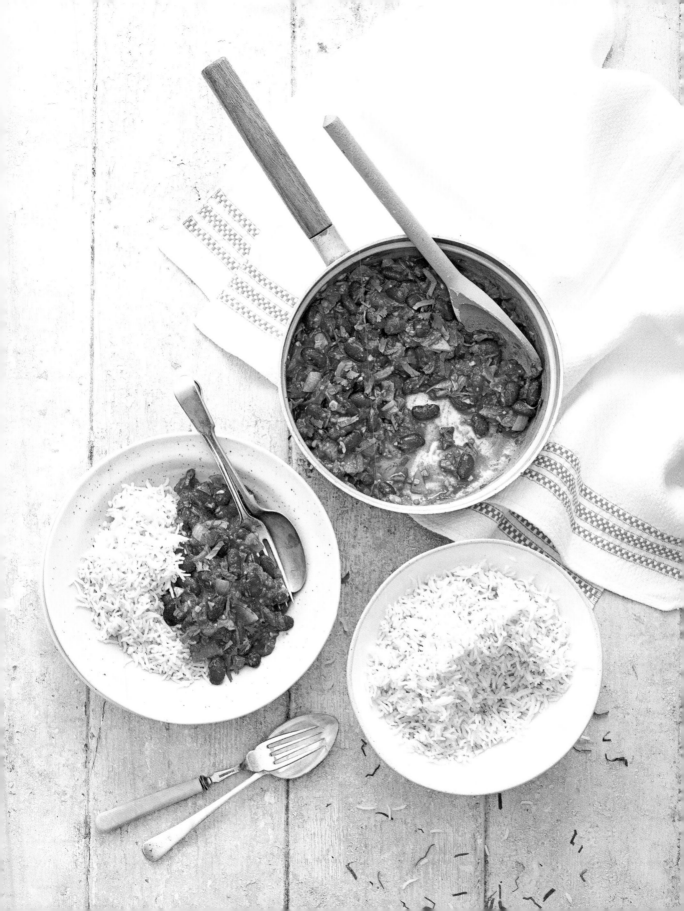

Microwave bacon & bean casserole

Eating alone doesn't have to mean boring baked beans on toast – turn them into a rich stew instead in under 15 minutes.

PREP 10 mins COOK 3 mins | 1

- 1 fat garlic clove, crushed
- 50g onion, chopped
- 1 tbsp olive oil
- 50g streaky bacon, diced
- ½ carrot, finely sliced or grated
- ¼ tsp mixed dried herbs, or a little fresh thyme or rosemary
- 100g baked beans
- 1 tbsp tomato purée
- ¼ chicken stock cube

1 In a microwaveable bowl, toss together the garlic and onion in the oil with a small pinch of salt. Add the bacon and microwave on High for 30–40 secs to soften the onion and garlic, and gently crisp the bacon. Tip in the carrot, herbs, baked beans and tomato purée, along with 1 tbsp water. Crumble over the stock cube and stir well.

2 Cover with cling film and pierce in the centre. Microwave on High for 2½ mins to heat through, then remove and stir well. Leave to stand for 1 min before serving.

Nutrition: *per serving*
kcal 444 fat 26g saturates 6g carbs 29g sugars 17g fibre 10g protein 20g salt 4.5g

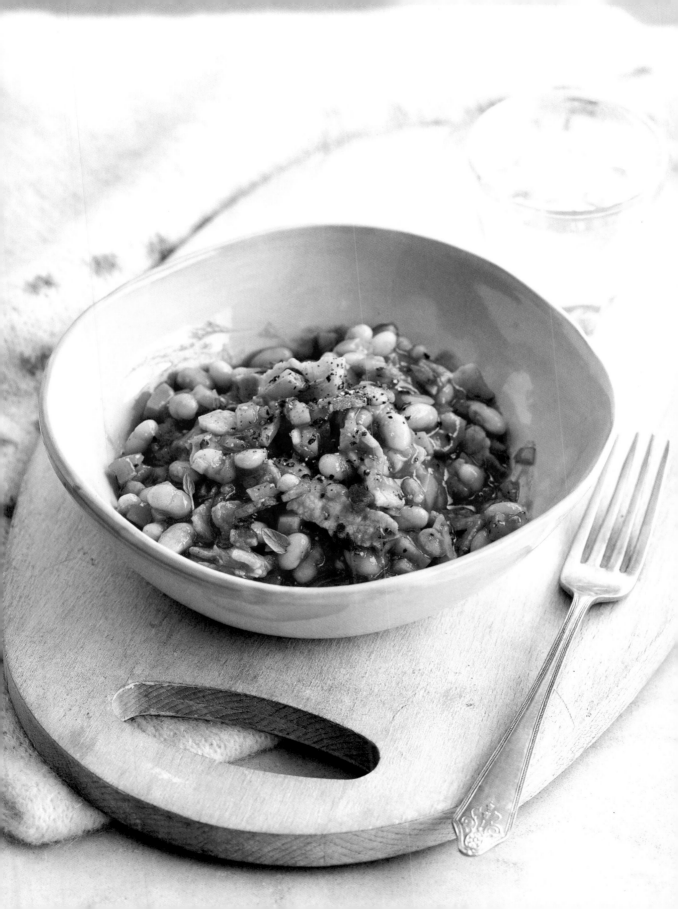

Sticky baked meatloaf with avocado & black bean salsa

A healthy and satisfying family supper with lean turkey mince and protein-packed quinoa, with a sticky onion glaze.

PREP 25 mins COOK 1 hr 15 mins 4

FOR THE MEATLOAF
- 1 tbsp rapeseed oil, plus a little for greasing
- 2 large onions, halved and thinly sliced
- 4 large garlic cloves, grated
- 1 tsp allspice or mixed spice
- 1½ tsp fennel seeds
- 2 tbsp smoked paprika
- 2 tbsp tomato purée
- 50g quinoa
- 160g grated carrot
- 1 tsp dried oregano
- ½ tsp ground cumin
- 400g pack turkey leg and breast mince
- 1 large egg
- 1 tsp black treacle

FOR THE SALSA
- 400g can black beans
- 1 small red onion, finely chopped
- 1 avocado, peeled, stoned and finely chopped
- 2 tomatoes, finely chopped
- ½ small pack coriander, chopped
- 1 red chilli, deseeded and finely chopped (optional)
- juice 1 lime

1 Heat oven to 180C/160C fan/gas 4. Grease and line a deep 500g loaf tin with baking parchment. Heat the oil in a large, non-stick frying pan. Add the onions and fry for 10 mins, stirring occasionally until golden. Stir in the garlic and spices, toast over the heat for 3 mins, then add the purée. Scrape half into a small bowl for the topping.

2 Stir the quinoa and 4 tbsp water into the frying pan and cook for 2 mins. Tip into a bowl, leave to cool for 5 mins, then add the carrot, oregano, cumin, turkey mince and egg. Season with black pepper and mix well. Pack into the greased tin and bake, uncovered, for 35 mins until firm.

3 Meanwhile, mix all the salsa ingredients in a serving bowl, and add 3 tbsp water to the remaining onion mixture with the black treacle.

4 When the meatloaf is cooked, carefully turn it out of the tin onto a shallow ovenproof dish and spread the onion mixture over the top. Return to the oven, bake for 10 mins more, then slice and serve with the salsa.

Nutrition: *per serving*
kcal 425 fat 13g saturates 3g carbs 31g sugars 15g fibre 14g protein 33g salt 0.6g

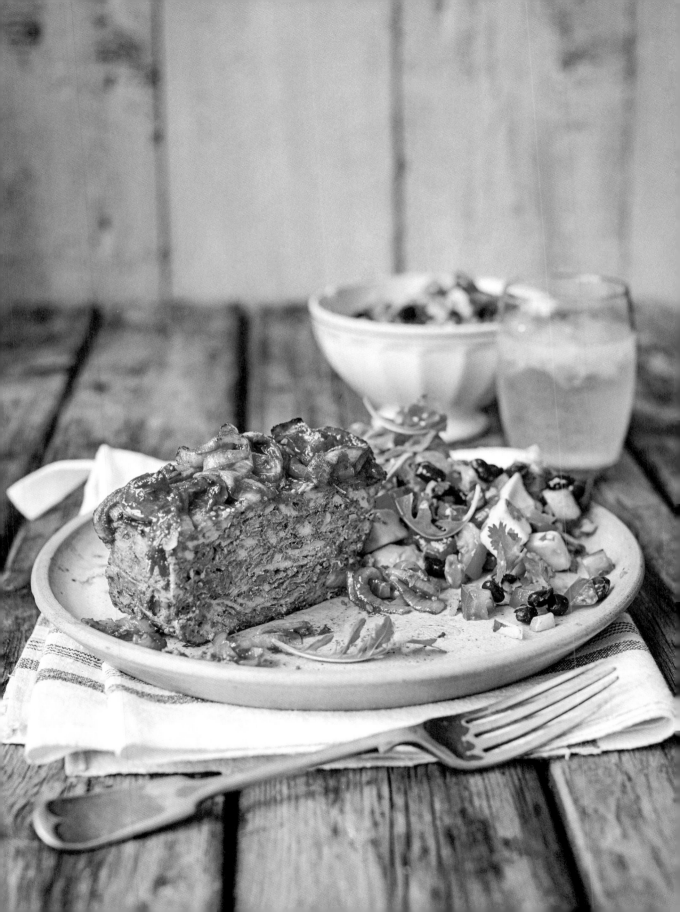

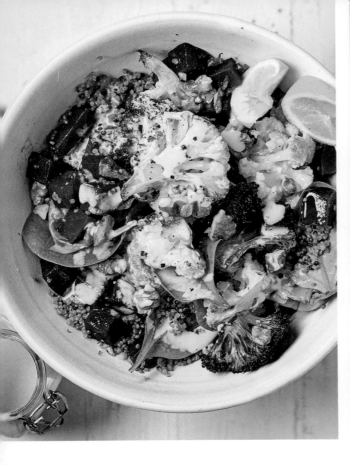
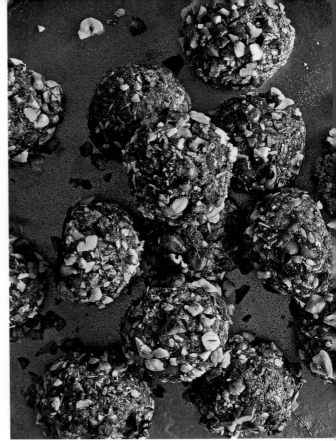
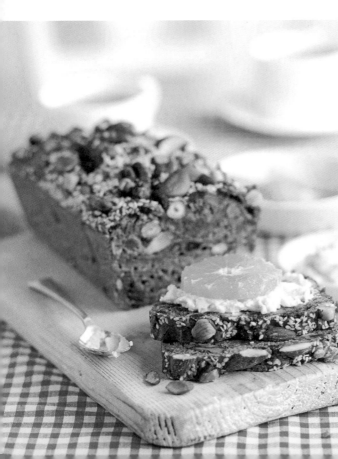
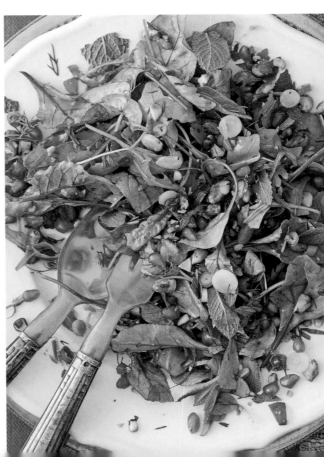

Chapter 6:

NUTS & SEEDS

· ·

These little superfoods punch well above their weight when it comes to nutritional bounty! We've used them both as the main component of a recipe like the almonds in our Ajo blanco (page 242) as well as a finishing flourish in our Porridge with beetroot, apple, cranberry compote & toasted hazelnuts (page 258).

Nuts and seeds make a fabulous addition to your diet, helping to top up levels of valuable minerals that can sometimes be difficult to obtain. Our Spicy seed mix (page 252) includes both sunflower and pumpkin seeds – sunflower seeds are one of the richest sources of magnesium and supply calcium and iron. Pumpkin seeds are rich in the protective mineral zinc, and supply more protein than most other seeds.

Full of fibre and one of the richest plant-sources of omega-3 fats, chia seeds help stabilize blood sugar levels and support brain function. They make a smart cooking ingredient because not only are they incredibly good for you they're also very versatile. In our Raw strawberry jam (page 252) we've used them as a thickener – this means we've been able to slash the sugar dramatically and create an altogether healthier toast topping! Another mighty seed is flaxseed – full of lignans, these little seeds help manage cholesterol and balance hormones, making them an invaluable dietary inclusion at the menopause and beyond.

Adding nut butter or tahini enriches a recipe by topping up levels of calcium, iron and zinc but also adds flavour, creaminess and texture. Try our delicious Black tahini chocolate cookies (page 254) – the black seeds are even richer in minerals than regular sesame seeds!

Lemon & marjoram sardines with walnut & pepper dressing

This is the ultimate recipe for glowing skin, packed with nutrients like calcium, vitamin C and heart-healthy omega-3 fats.

⏱ PREP 25 mins COOK 5 mins 🍽 2

- 6 butterflied sardines
- 2 garlic cloves, crushed
- juice and zest 1 lemon
- 2 tsp marjoram or oregano, plus a few extra leaves for sprinkling
- generous handful walnut halves
- 100g roasted red peppers from a jar (not in oil), drained
- small drizzle extra virgin rapeseed oil
- baby spinach leaves
- seeds from ½ pomegranate

1 Open up the sardines and smear the flesh with half the garlic. Grate over the lemon zest (reserving a little to serve) and season with black pepper. Scatter over half the marjoram or oregano, then close the sardines again.

2 Put the walnuts, remaining herbs and the peppers in a bowl. Season, then blitz to a rough purée with a blender. Add the remaining garlic and a generous squeeze of lemon from one half, and blitz again.

3 Heat a drop of oil in a large non-stick frying pan and quickly wilt the spinach, then set aside. Wipe out the pan, then heat a little more oil and cook the sardines for 2 mins each side. Arrange the spinach on 2 plates and top with the sardines, scatter over the pomegranate seeds, then top with the dressing. Sprinkle over the reserved lemon zest and a few herb leaves, then serve with the remaining half of the lemon, cut into wedges.

Nutrition: *per serving*
kcal 335 fat 17g saturates 3g carbs 14g sugars 10g fibre 6g protein 27g salt 0.7g

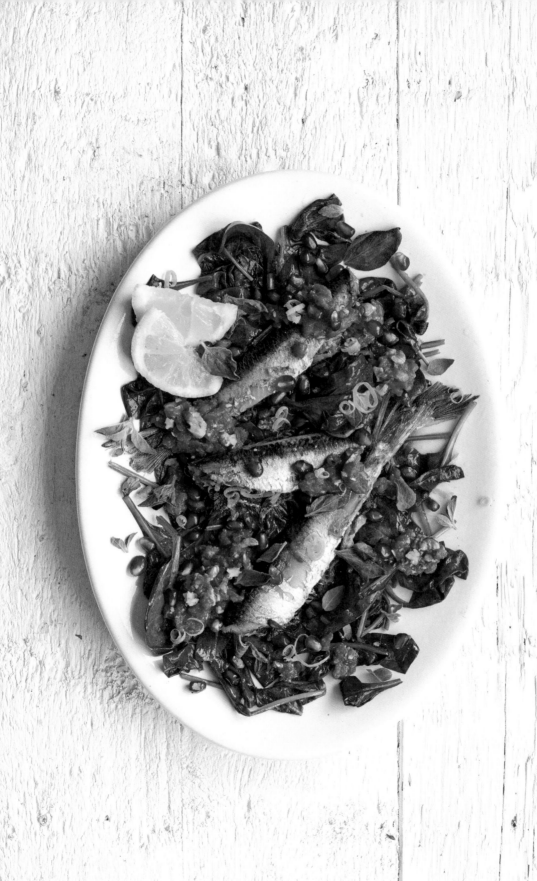

Roasted cauli-broc bowl with tahini houmous

A simple quinoa bowl you can put together in 10 minutes and enjoy al-desko. It's vegan, healthy and gluten-free.

🕐 PREP 10 mins COOK 30 mins 🥧 2

- 400g pack cauliflower & broccoli florets
- 2 tbsp olive oil
- 250g ready-to-eat quinoa
- 2 cooked beetroots, cubed
- large handful baby spinach
- 10 walnuts, toasted and chopped
- 2 tbsp tahini
- 3 tbsp houmous
- 1 lemon, ½ juiced, ½ cut into wedges

1 Heat oven to 200C/180C fan/gas 6. Put the cauliflower and broccoli in a large roasting tin with the oil and a sprinkle of flaky sea salt. Roast for 25–30 mins until browned and cooked. Leave to cool completely.

2 Build each bowl by putting half the quinoa in each. Lay the slices of beetroot on top, followed by the spinach, cauliflower, broccoli and walnuts. Combine the tahini, houmous, lemon juice and 1 tbsp water in a small pot. Before eating, coat in the dressing. Serve with the lemon wedges.

Nutrition: *per serving*
kcal 533 fat 37g saturates 4g carbs 28g sugars 6g fibre 10g protein 16g salt 0.8g

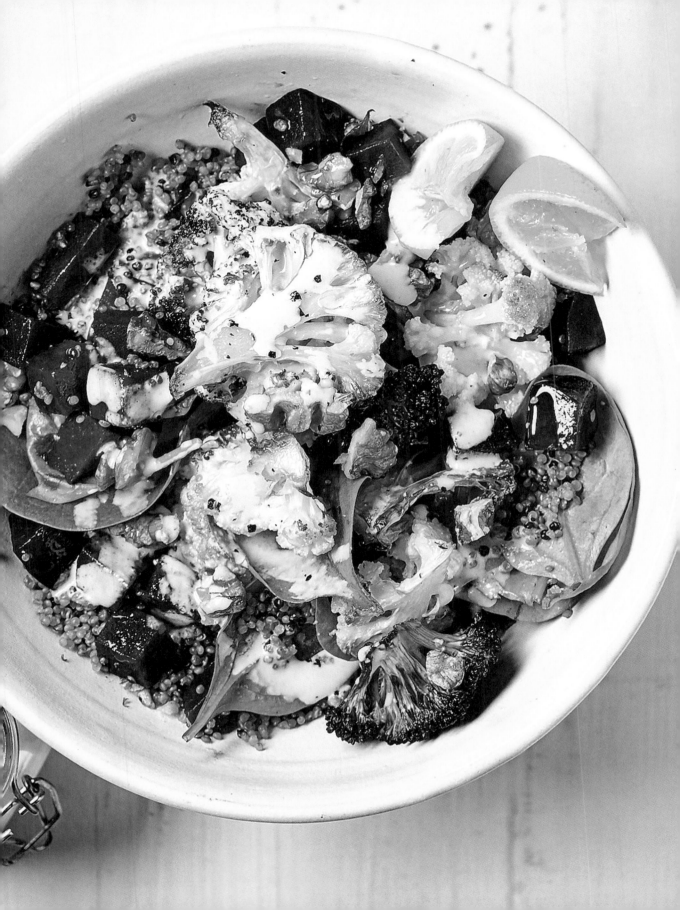

Triple nut & apple stuffing balls

These vegetarian red onion, lentil and sage stuffing balls are packed with texture from crunchy linseeds, pecans, hazelnuts and pistachios – a welcome addition to any Sunday lunch.

🕐 PREP 20 mins COOK 30 mins 🥧 16

- 2 tbsp linseeds
- 1 red onion, halved
- 1 tbsp olive oil, plus extra for greasing
- 200g mixed nuts of your choice (we used a combination of pecans, hazelnuts and pistachios)
- 400g can cooked green lentils in water, drained
- 50g wholemeal breadcrumbs
- small bunch sage, chopped
- 1 small apple, grated

1 Put the linseeds in a small bowl and mix with 2 tbsp water, then set aside for 5–10 mins until the water thickens to a gluey consistency. Meanwhile, place the onion in a food processor and whizz until finely chopped. Heat the oil in a frying pan, tip in the onion and cook for 5 mins until softened.

2 Tip the nuts into the food processor and whizz until coarsely chopped. Sprinkle 3 tbsp of the nuts over a plate and set aside. Add the lentils, breadcrumbs, sage, apple, linseeds (and any liquid in the bowl), onion and plenty of seasoning to the processor. Pulse to blend the mixture until just combined – don't chop too finely or the stuffing will lose its nice nutty texture.

3 Line a baking tray with foil and grease with a little oil. Remove the blade from the processor and oil your hands. Scoop out walnut-sized chunks of stuffing, roll into balls, then roll on the plate of chopped nuts to coat. Place on the prepared baking tray. Can be covered with cling film and chilled for up to 2 days, or frozen for 2 months.

4 Heat oven to 200C/180C fan/gas 6. Unwrap (if chilled) and bake for 25–30 mins until the nuts are a little darker and the balls have firmed up slightly – they will be softer than traditional stuffing balls but will firm up after a few mins cooling. If you're cooking from frozen, bake for 35–40 mins.

Nutrition: *per ball*
kcal 119 fat 9g saturates 1g carbs 5g sugars 2g fibre 2g protein 3g salt 0g

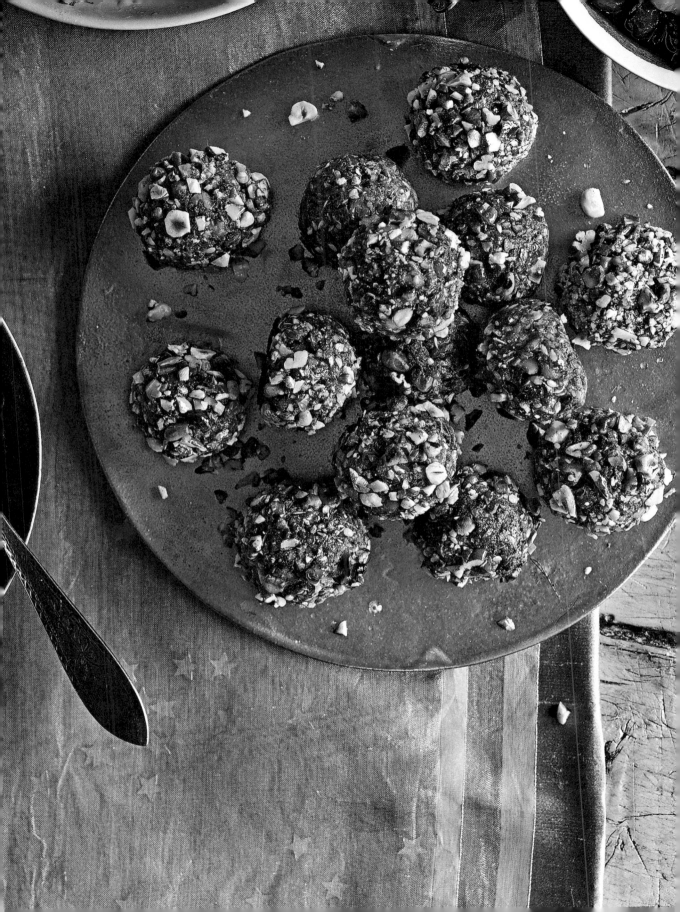

Fennel, walnut, cherry & goat's cheese salad

This seasonal salad is packed with contrasting flavours and textures such as crunchy walnuts, hearty Puy lentils and juicy cherries.

PREP 15 mins COOK 5 mins 2-3

- 50g walnut halves or pieces
- 250g pack pre-cooked Puy lentils
- 1 large fennel bulb, finely sliced, fronds reserved
- 140g cherries, halved and pitted (or small figs, halved)
- 1 tbsp red wine vinegar
- 2 tbsp extra virgin olive oil
- 1 tsp Dijon mustard
- ½ tsp clear honey
- ½ small pack tarragon, roughly chopped
- 100g pack soft goat's cheese, thickly sliced and halved

1 Heat a dry frying pan over a low-medium heat. Add the walnuts and cook for 3 mins, stirring frequently, until they smell toasty and the skins are a deep golden brown. Set aside to cool.
2 Heat the lentils following pack instructions, then tip into a large bowl and loosen with a fork. Tip the fennel and cherries on top.
3 Whisk together the vinegar, oil, mustard, honey and tarragon, then season. Fold the dressing through the lentils, fennel and cherries, then scoop the salad onto a platter. Scatter with the cheese, walnuts and the reserved fennel fronds.

Nutrition: *per serving (3)*
kcal 466 fat 29g saturates 8g carbs 26g sugars 9g fibre 10g protein 20g salt 1.6g

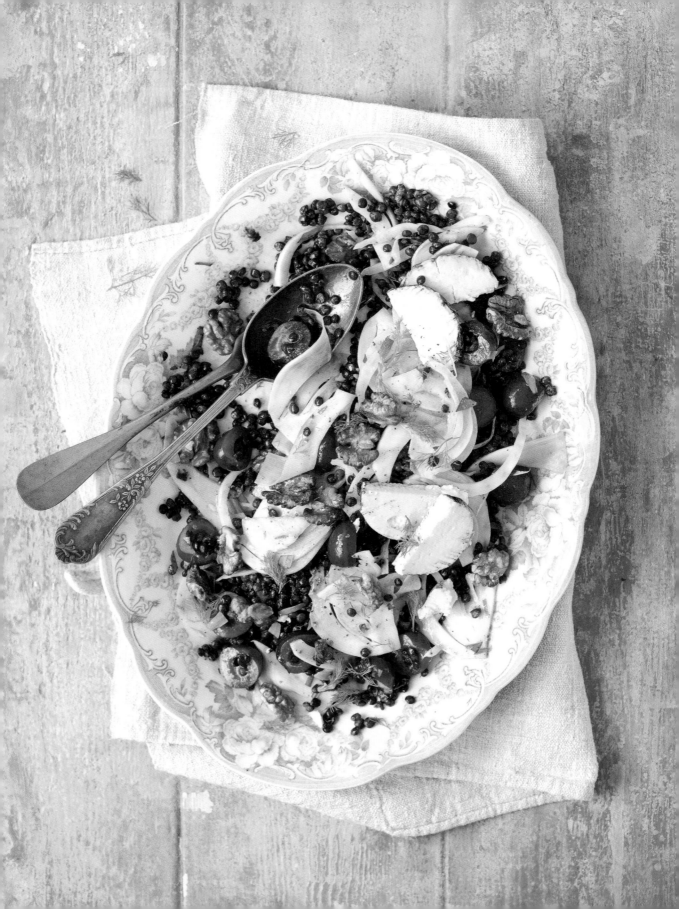

Almond butter, goji berry & banana tartine

· ·

These nutty banana and berry toasts will keep you going all morning – sweet, simple and super quick to make.

🕐 PREP 5 mins COOK 5 mins 🥧 2

- 4 slices of your favourite bread (we used sourdough)
- 4 tbsp almond butter
- 1 banana, cut into thin rounds
- 1 tbsp goji berries
- ½ tbsp sunflower seeds
- drizzle of honey

Toast the bread, then top with the almond butter, banana, goji berries and sunflower seeds. Drizzle over the honey and sprinkle with some flaky sea salt.

· ·

Nutrition: *per serving*
kcal 607 fat 22g saturates 2g carbs 77g sugars 21g fibre 8g protein 22g salt 1.4g

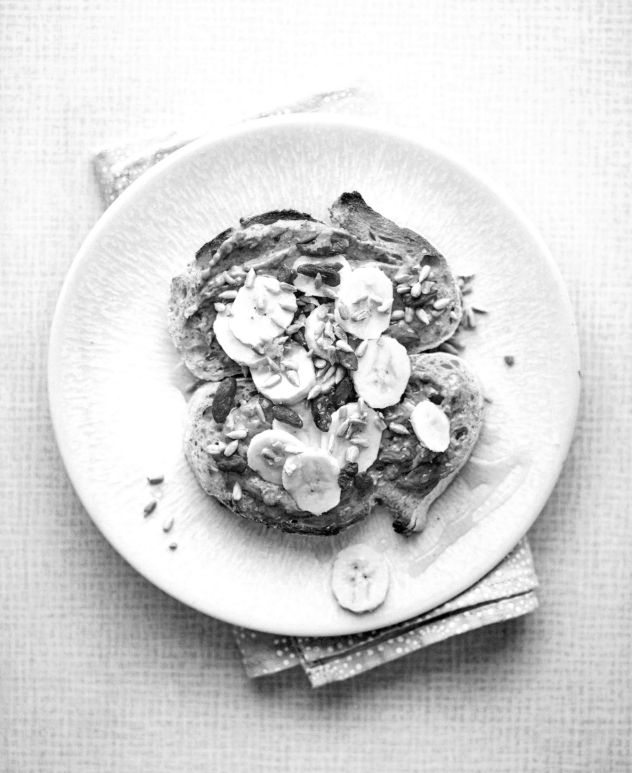

Ajo blanco

· ·

This authentic chilled Spanish soup can be made ahead and stored in the fridge for up to 3 days.

🕐 PREP 5 mins plus chilling NO COOK 🥧 2

- 200g blanched almonds
- 50ml extra virgin olive oil
- 1 garlic clove
- 1½ tbsp red wine vinegar

Blend the ingredients together with 350ml water and 1 tsp salt. Let the soup chill in the fridge for 1 hr or so, then serve with a drizzle of oil and some black pepper.

· ·

Nutrition: *per serving*
kcal 265 fat 25g saturates 3g carbs 2g sugars 1g fibre 0g protein 8g salt 0.8g

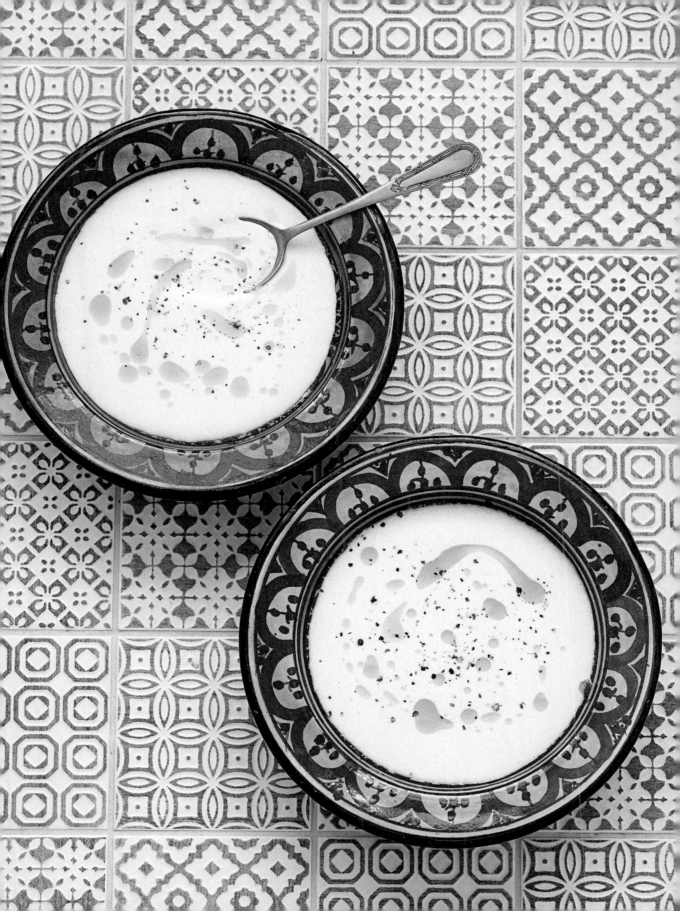

Almond, cashew & honey butter

Homemade nut butters are packed with vitamins and minerals. Spread this on sourdough toast or blend in a smoothie.

PREP 10 mins Cook time 10 mins 1 jar

- 200g blanched almonds
- 200g unsalted cashew nuts
- 2 tbsp honey
- ½ tsp sea salt flakes
- 2–3 tsp groundnut oil

1 Heat oven to 200C/180C fan/gas 6. Tip the nuts onto a large baking tray, place in the oven and roast for 10 mins, stirring now and then to ensure they don't catch at the edges. When golden brown, remove from the oven and leave to cool completely.

2 Tip the nuts into a food processor, add the honey and salt. Blend for 8–9 mins, until you're left with a smooth nut butter. If you want to loosen the consistency, add a drizzle of oil and blend again.

Nutrition: per tbsp
kcal 88 fat 7g saturates 1g carbs 3g sugars 2g fibre 0.3g protein 3g salt 0.1g

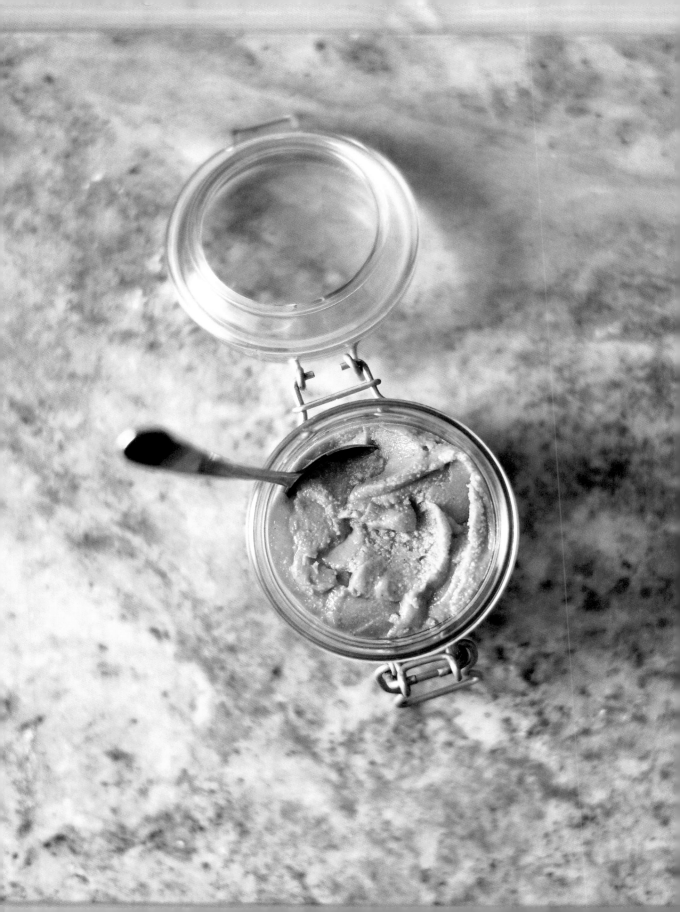

Light chicken korma

The whole family will love this mild, creamy curry.

PREP 10 mins COOK 25 mins | 4

- 1 onion, chopped
- 2 garlic cloves, roughly chopped
- thumb-sized piece ginger, roughly chopped
- 4 tbsp korma paste
- 4 skinless, boneless chicken breasts cut into bite-sized pieces
- 50g ground almonds
- 4 tbsp sultanas
- 400ml chicken stock
- ¼ tsp golden caster sugar
- 150g Greek yogurt
- small bunch coriander, chopped
- flaked almonds, to serve (optional)

1 Put the onion, garlic and ginger in a food processor and whizz to a paste. Tip the paste into a large high-sided frying pan with 3 tbsp water and cook for 5 mins. Add the korma paste and cook for a further 2 mins until aromatic.

2 Stir the chicken into the sauce, then add the ground almonds, sultanas, stock and sugar. Give everything a good mix, then cover and simmer for 10 mins or until the chicken is cooked through.

3 Remove the pan from the heat, stir in the yogurt and some seasoning, then scatter over the coriander and flaked almonds, if using. Serve with brown or white basmati rice.

Nutrition: *per serving*
kcal 398 fat 12g saturates 2g carbs 29g sugars 27g fibre 4g protein 40g salt 1.1g

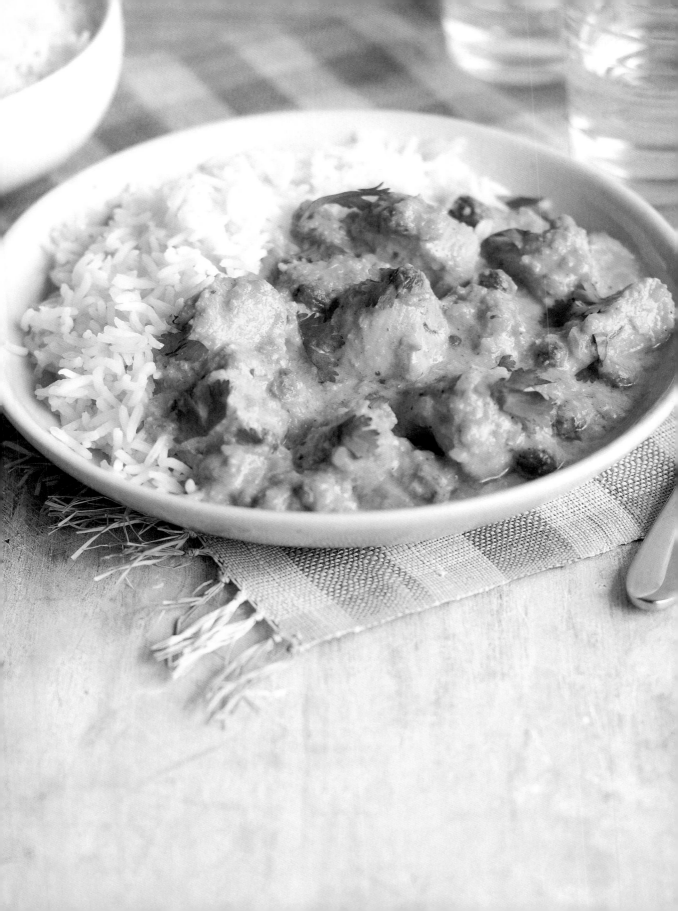

Fig, nut & seed bread

This healthy bread is packed with goodness. Make a loaf and eat over a week, topped with nut butter, jam, ricotta or fresh fruit.

🕐 PREP 15 mins COOK 1 hr 15 mins 🥧 16

- 400ml hot strong black tea
- 100g dried figs, hard stalks removed, thinly sliced
- 140g sultanas
- 50g porridge oats
- 200g self-raising wholemeal flour
- 1 tsp baking powder
- 100g mixed nuts (almonds, walnuts, Brazils, hazelnuts), plus 50g for the topping
- 1 tbsp golden linseed
- 1 tbsp sesame seeds, plus 2 tsp to sprinkle
- 25g pumpkin seeds
- 1 large egg
- ricotta and sliced orange to serve, optional

1 Heat oven to 170C/150C fan/gas 3½. Pour the tea into a large bowl and stir in the figs, sultanas and oats. Set aside to soak.
2 Meanwhile, line the base and sides of a 1kg loaf tin with baking parchment. Mix together the flour, baking powder, nuts and seeds. Beat the egg into the cooled fruit mixture, then stir the dry ingredients into the wet. Pour into the tin, then level the top and scatter with the extra nuts and sesame seeds.
3 Bake for 1 hr, then cover the top with foil and bake for 15 mins more until a skewer inserted into the centre of the loaf comes out clean. Remove from the tin to cool, but leave the parchment on until cold. Will keep in the fridge for 1 month, or freeze in slices.

Nutrition: *per serving (1 slice with 25g ricotta and fruit)*
kcal 249 fat 10g saturates 3g carbs 30g sugars 20g fibre 6g protein 10g salt 0.3g

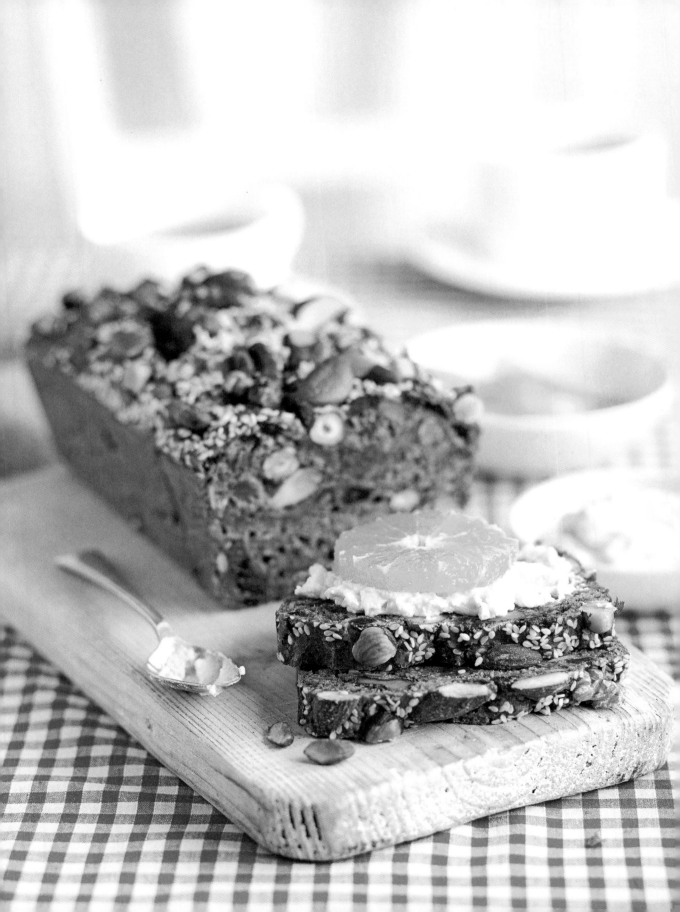

Breakfast bars

This fruity, chewy flapjack is packed with delicious oats and cereal - kids can help make them and they're perfect for lunchboxes.

🕐 PREP 20 mins COOK 25 mins 🥧 10

- 50g mixed dried fruit (a mixture of raisins, sultanas and apricots is nice)
- 50g mixed seeds
- 140g oats
- 25g multi-grain hoop cereal
- 100g butter
- 100g light muscovado sugar
- 100g golden syrup

1 Grease and line a 20cm square cake tin with baking parchment. Put the dried fruit in a mixing bowl. Add the seeds, oats and cereal, and mix well.

2 Put the butter, sugar and golden syrup in the saucepan. Cook gently on the hob, stirring with the spatula, until the butter and sugar are melted. Remove from the heat and pour the dry ingredients into the saucepan. Mix well until all the ingredients are coated with the syrup mix.

3 Fill the baking tin with the mixture. Use the spatula to press the mix down evenly. Bake at 160C/140C fan/gas 3 for 20 mins, then leave to cool completely before cutting into squares or fingers. Store in an airtight tin for up to 3 days – if they last that long!

Nutrition: *per bar*
kcal 205 fat 10g saturates 5g carbs 25g sugars 17g fibre 2g protein 3g salt 0.2g

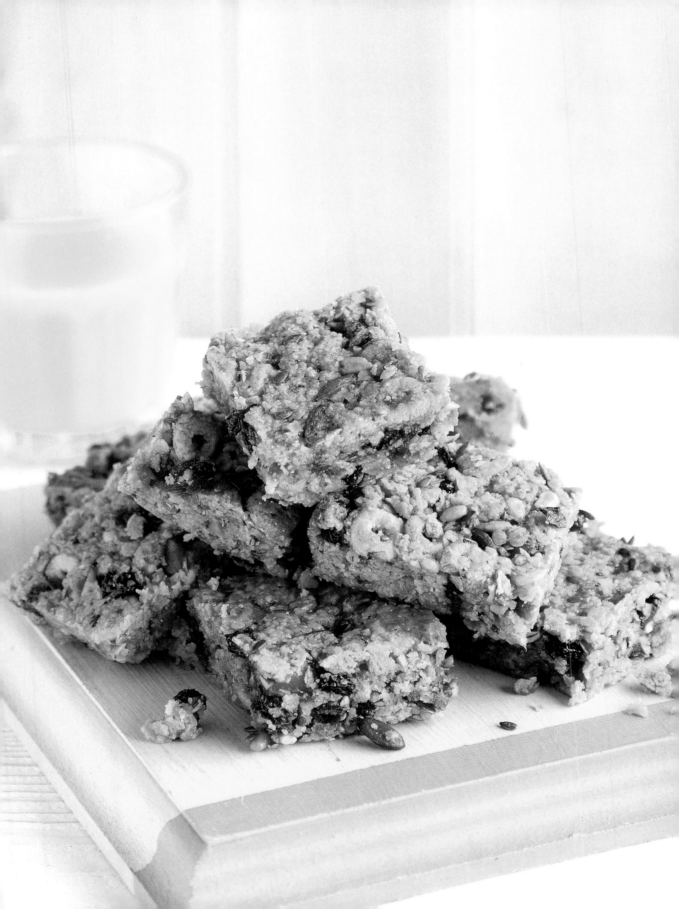

Raw strawberry jam

Chia seeds work their magic in this no-cook jam. Within minutes of being mixed with the strawberry pulp they will thicken it, meaning there's no need to boil it or add jam sugar. It won't last as long as regular jam, so use up within 4 days.

PREP 1 hour 5 mins NO COOK   1 X 350g jar

- 400g strawberries, hulled
- 2 tbsp lemon juice
- 2 tbsp maple syrup
- 2 tbsp chia seeds

Blend 3/4 of the strawberries and roughly chop the rest. Add the rest of the ingredients, mix well and leave for 1 hr, stirring occasionally, until thickened. Store in a sterilised jar in the fridge for up to 4 days or freeze for up to 1 month.

Nutrition: *per tbsp*
kcal 12 fat 0.3g saturates 0g carbs 2g sugars 1g fibre 1g protein 0.2g salt 0g

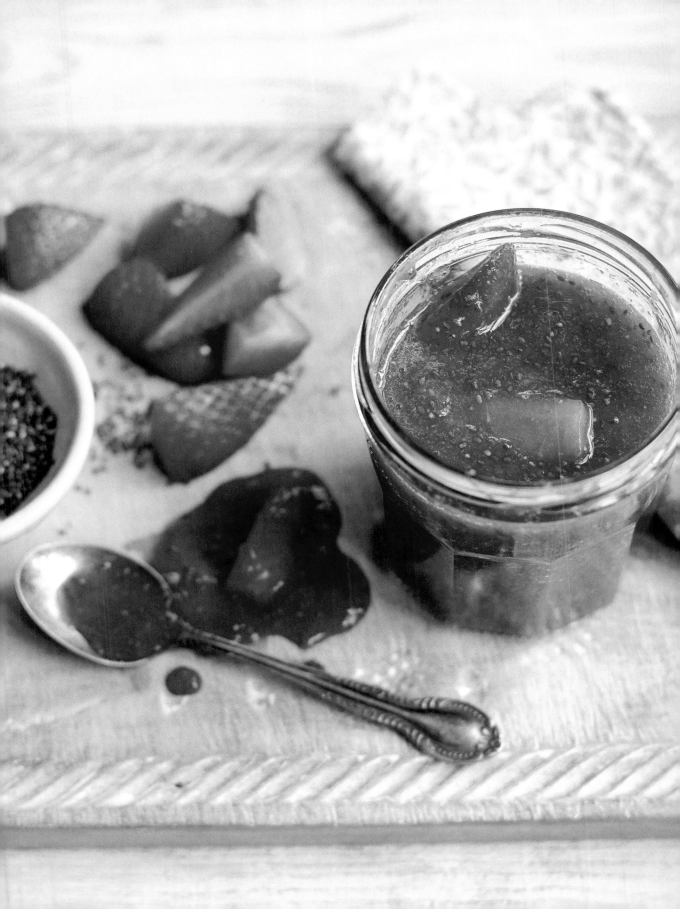

Black tahini chocolate cookies

Treat yourself to these delicious cookies, in the knowledge they're doing you some good. Tahini is rich in minerals such as potassium, magnesium and iron.

PREP 20 mins COOK 8 mins 20

- 50g salted butter, softened
- 125g light brown muscovado sugar
- 125g golden caster sugar
- 1 egg, beaten
- 200g self-raising flour
- 2 tbsp cocoa powder
- 200g milk chocolate, broken into chunks
- 100g white chocolate, melted, for drizzling

FOR THE BLACK TAHINI
- 100g black sesame seeds, plus extra for decorating
- 100g flavourless oil
- 30ml maple syrup

1 First, make the black tahini. Toast the sesame seeds in a small pan over a gentle heat until you can smell the sesame aroma. Transfer to a mini processor and blitz. Pour in the oil gradually until a paste forms. Add the maple syrup and blitz again. Tip into a small bowl until ready to use.

2 Heat oven to 180C/160C fan/gas 4 and line 2 baking sheets with parchment. In a large bowl, beat the butter and sugars together until pale and fluffy. Add the egg and 80g of black tahini paste, and beat to combine. Tip in the flour, cocoa and milk chocolate chunks, and beat until fully incorporated.

3 Using an ice cream scoop, ball the dough into about 20 pieces and place on the baking sheets. Press each ball lightly so it's a little flatter, leaving plenty of room between them, as they will spread.

4 Bake for 6–8 mins until still soft in the middle – they will harden as they cool. Leave to cool on the sheets for a few mins before transferring to wire racks to cool completely.

5 Once cooled, drizzle white chocolate zigzags all over the cookies and sprinkle some black sesame seeds on top. Will keep in an airtight container for 3 days.

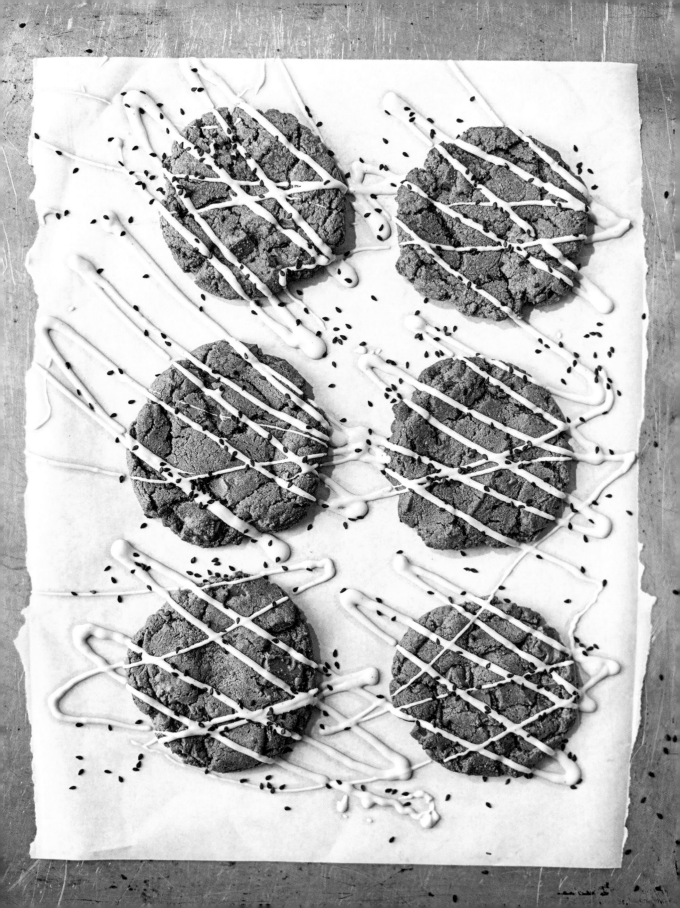

Raspberry ripple chia pudding

Fancy raspberry ripple for breakfast? Well now you can with our vegan chia pudding bowl.

PREP 10 mins NO COOK · 2

- 50g white chia seeds
- 200ml coconut drinking milk
- 1 nectarine or peach, cut into slices
- 2 tbsp goji berries

FOR THE RASPBERRY PURÉE
- 100g raspberries
- 1 tsp lemon juice
- 2 tsp maple syrup

1 Divide the chia seeds and coconut milk between 2 serving bowls and stir well. Leave to soak for 5 mins, stirring occasionally, until the seeds swell and thicken when stirred.

2 Meanwhile, combine the purée ingredients in a small food processor, or blitz with a hand blender. Swirl a spoonful into each bowl, then arrange the nectarine or peach slices on top and scatter with the goji berries. Will keep in the fridge for 1 day. Add the toppings just before serving.

Nutrition: *per serving*
kcal 257 fat 10g saturates 3g carbs 26g sugars 22g fibre 13g protein 8g salt 0.2g

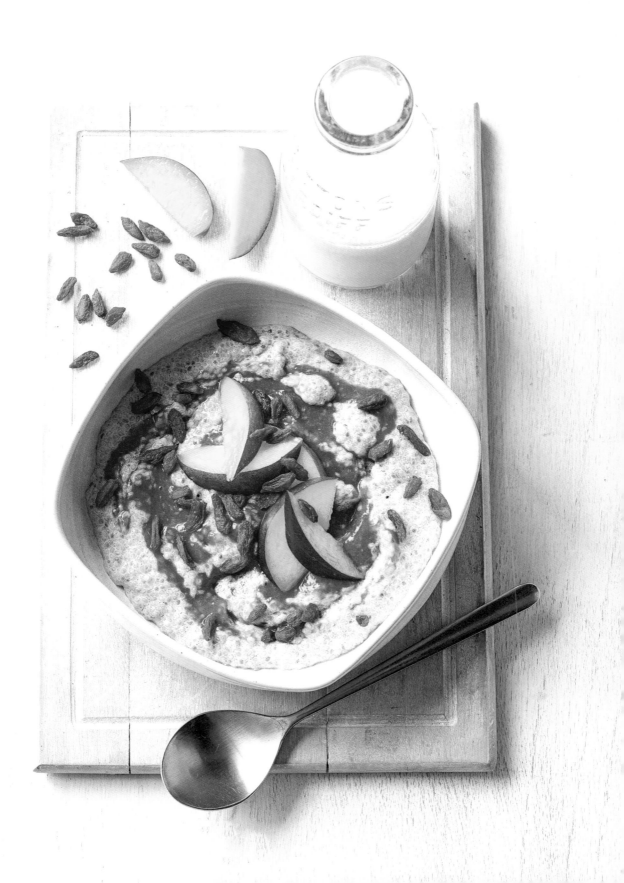

Porridge with beetroot, apple, cranberry compote & toasted hazelnuts

Finish creamy oats with a subtly spiced, fruity topping of cinnamon, cardamom and maple syrup for a warming breakfast or weekend brunch.

PREP 10 mins plus soaking COOK 35 mins 2

- 100g oats, soaked overnight in in 250ml water (for best texture, use an equal combination of porridge oats and jumbo oats)
- 250ml almond milk, coconut milk or full-fat milk
- pinch of flaked sea salt

FOR THE COMPOTE
- 1 eating apple, core removed and diced
- 140g cranberries, fresh or frozen
- 1 raw beetroot, coarsely grated
- 2 tbsp maple syrup
- 75ml orange juice
- 1 tsp ground cinnamon
- ¼ tsp vanilla extract
- cardamom pods (seeds only, pounded using a pestle and mortar)

TO SERVE
- 2 tbsp Greek yogurt or coconut yogurt
- handful hazelnuts, toasted and chopped

1 Put all the compote ingredients in a saucepan over a medium heat and bring to the boil, then lower to a simmer for 30 mins, adding a little water, 1 tbsp at a time, if needed.

2 Once the compote is cooked, put the soaked oats, milk and a good pinch of flaked sea salt in a saucepan, and warm over a medium heat for 3–4 mins.

3 Divide the porridge between 2 bowls, add a heaped tbsp of compote, the yogurt and a scattering of crushed hazelnuts, to serve.

Nutrition: *per serving*
kcal 338 fat 5g saturates 1g carbs 57g sugars 25g fibre 11g protein 10g salt 0.2g

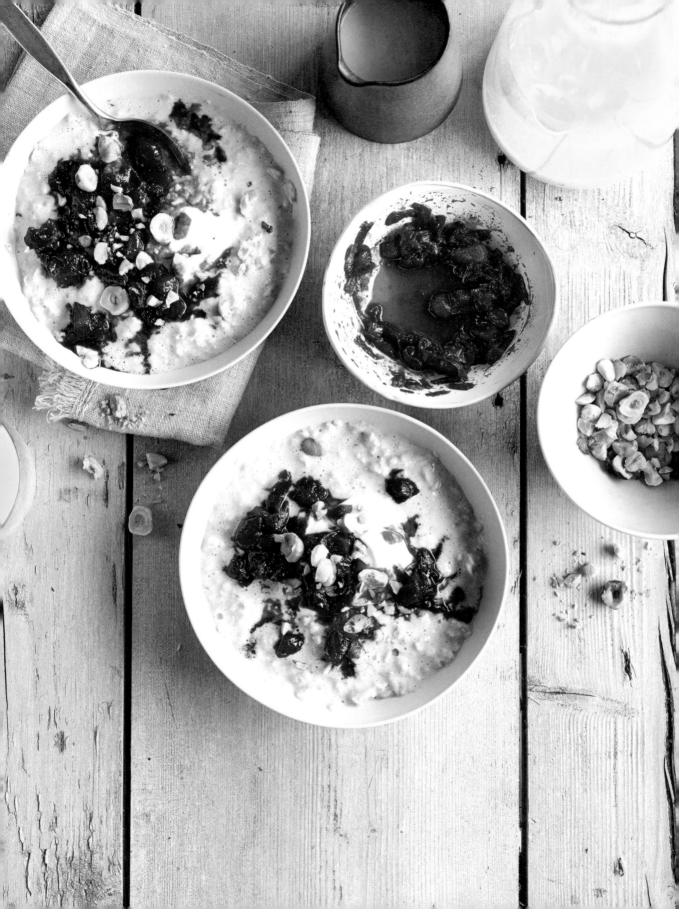

Herb salad with pomegranate & pistachios

Serve this herby salad with lamb cutlets for a special dinner.

🕐 PREP 15 mins NO COOK 🥧 6

- juice 1 orange
- 3 tbsp red wine vinegar
- 1 tbsp clear honey
- small bunch dill, very roughly chopped
- small bunch mint, picked and torn
- bunch spring onions, finely sliced
- 100g bag mixed salad leaves
- 120g tub pomegranate seeds (or seeds from 1 pomegranate)
- 100g bag pistachios, roughly chopped

Mix the juice, vinegar and honey with seasoning. Tip rest of the ingredients into a large mixing bowl, drizzle over the dressing and gently toss to serve.

Nutrition: *per serving*
kcal 131 fat 9g saturates 1g carbs 8g sugars 8g fibre 1g protein 4g salt 0.01g

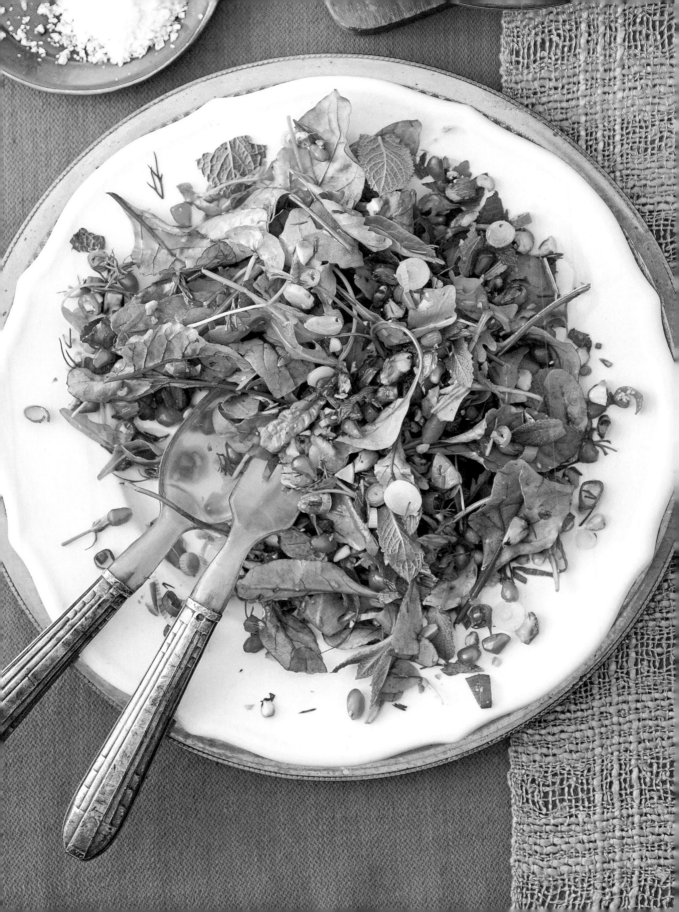

Pistachio & cardamom butter

A storecupboard twist on traditional nut butters, with moreish pistachios and cardamom pods.

PREP 10 mins NO COOK 1 jar

- 10 cardamom pods
- 400g pistachio nut kernels
- 1 tbsp maple syrup
- ½ tsp sea salt flakes
- 2–3 tsp groundnut oil

1 Remove the seeds from the cardamom pods and finely crush them in a pestle and mortar.
2 Tip the nuts into a food processor, add the crushed cardamom, maple syrup and salt. Blend for 7–8 mins, until you're left with a smooth nut butter. To loosen the consistency, add a drizzle of oil and blend again.

Nutrition: *per tbsp*
kcal 87 fat 7g saturates 1g carbs 3g sugars 1g fibre 2g protein 3g salt 0.1g

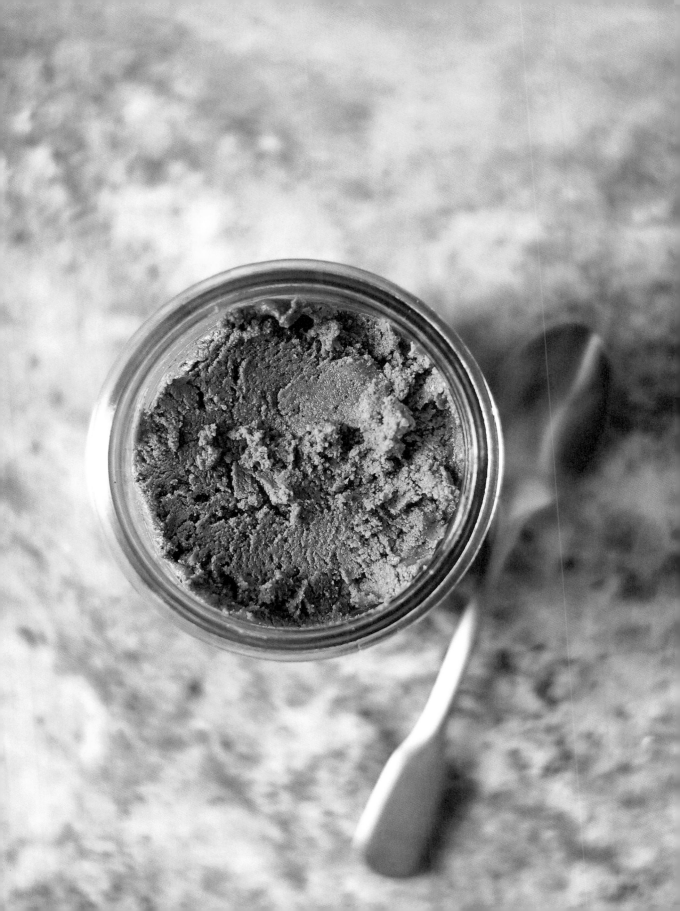

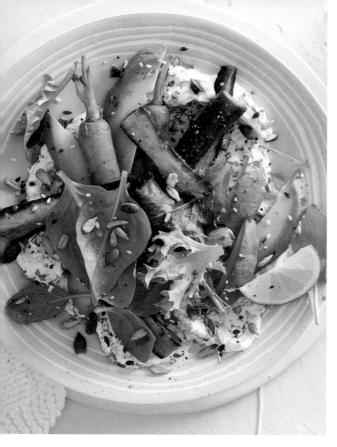
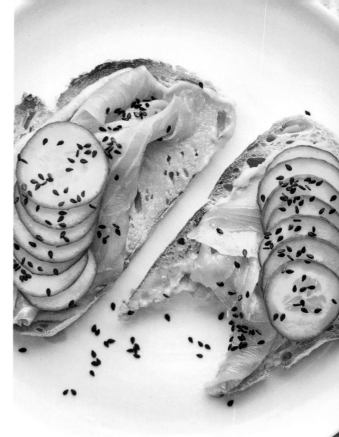
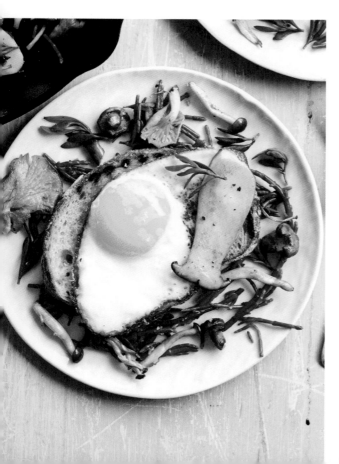
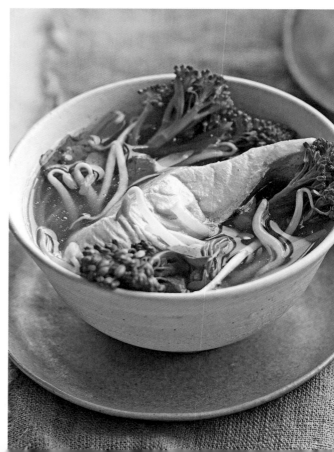

Chapter 7:

FERMENTED FOODS

· ·

'Live' yogurt, kefir and fermented foods like kimchi, sauerkraut and miso help repopulate the gut with healthy, gut-friendly bacteria. These probiotic foods are important for maintaining the health of the gut, manufacturing certain vitamins and protecting the intestinal lining. It's said that 60–70% of our immune defences reside in the gut so protecting and maintaining a favourable environment here is crucial to fighting off those unwanted bugs. Add a small portion of fermented foods like kimchi or sauerkraut once or twice a day to improve digestion and strengthen your immunity.

We've used miso in our Miso brown rice & broccoli salad with prawns (page 266) – if you're unfamiliar with this Asian ingredient it's a paste made from fermented soya beans and is rich in these beneficial bacteria. Choose the naturally fermented and unpasteurized variety.

As well repopulating the gut with beneficial bacteria we also need to feed them in order to encourage their growth. It's prebiotic foods like onions, leeks and asparagus as well as oatmeal, bananas and legumes that make an important contribution here. Make these a plentiful addition to your regular diet.

Miso brown rice & broccoli salad with prawns

Fermented soya bean paste, miso, is high in beneficial bacteria. Stir leftover miso paste into stir-fries or make into a simple broth with hot stock or water.

PREP 15 mins COOK 25 mins 3

- 100g brown basmati rice
- 140g ready-shelled frozen edamame beans
- 140g broccoli (about ½ a head), broken into florets
- 1 tbsp white or brown miso paste
- ½ tsp finely grated fresh ginger
- 1 tbsp rice vinegar
- ½ tbsp clear honey
- 2 tsp sesame oil
- 2 tsp vegetable oil
- 3 garlic cloves, thinly sliced
- 1 red chilli, thinly sliced
- 200g raw shelled prawns
- 2 spring onions, finely sliced
- large pack coriander, roughly chopped

1 Cook the rice following pack instructions, adding the edamame beans for the last 3 mins of cooking. Drain well.

2 Meanwhile, steam the broccoli for 4–5 mins until tender. Run under very cold water, drain thoroughly and pat dry. In a small bowl, mix the miso, ginger, vinegar, honey, sesame oil and seasoning.

3 Heat the vegetable oil in a non-stick frying pan. Add the garlic and ½ the chilli and cook gently for a couple of mins, taking care not to burn. Throw in the prawns, lots of black pepper and a pinch of salt. Turn up the heat and cook for a few mins until the prawns are cooked through. Toss the miso dressing with the cooked rice, adding the spring onions, coriander and broccoli. Season and stir together. Spoon the spicy prawns on top, scatter over the remaining chilli and serve.

Nutrition: *per serving*
kcal 304 fat 8g saturates 1g carbs 35g sugars 6g fibre 5g protein 21g salt 0.6g

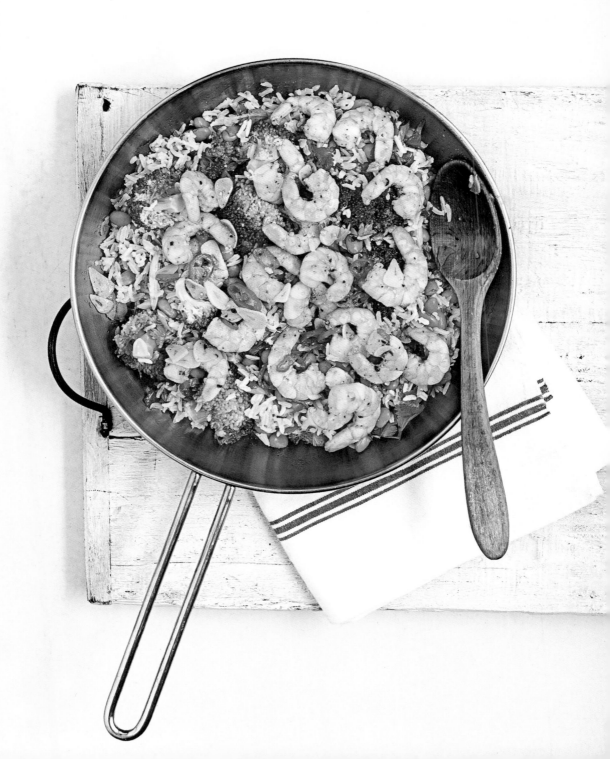

Simple sauerkraut

The simplest way to make classic sauerkraut – a fermented food that's great for your gut. It's extra tasty served with sausages and mustard.

PREP 30 mins plus fermenting NO COOK 4 x 450ml jars

- 2kg very firm, pale green or white cabbage (any leathery outer leaves removed), cored
- 3 tbsp coarse crystal sea salt (or 6 tbsp flaky sea salt)
- 1 tsp caraway seeds
- 1 tsp peppercorns

1 Thoroughly wash a large tub or bowl (about the size of a small washing-up bowl), then rinse with boiling water from the kettle. Make sure that your hands, and everything else coming into contact with the cabbage, are very clean. It's wise to use a container that will comfortably fit the softened cabbage, allowing several inches of room at the top to avoid overflow.

2 Shred the cabbage thinly – a food processor makes light work of this. Layer the cabbage and the salt in the tub or bowl. Massage the salt into the cabbage for 5 mins, wait 5 mins, then repeat. You should end up with a much-reduced volume of cabbage sitting in its own brine. Mix in the caraway seeds and the peppercorns.

3 Cover the surface of the cabbage entirely with a sheet of cling film, then press out all the air bubbles from below. Weigh the cabbage down using a couple of heavy plates, or other weights that fit your bowl, and cover as much of the cabbage as possible. The level of the brine will rise to cover the cabbage a little. Cover the tub with its lid (or more cling film) and leave in a dark place at a cool room temperature (about 18-20C) for at least 5 days. It will be ready to eat after 5 days, but for maximum flavour leave the cabbage to ferment for anywhere between 2–6 weeks (or until the bubbling subsides).

4 Check the cabbage every day or so, releasing any gases that have built up as it ferments, and give the cabbage a stir to release the bubbles. If any scum forms, remove it, rinse the weights in boiling water and replace the cling film. You should see bubbles appearing within the cabbage, and possibly some foam on the top of the brine. It's important to keep it at an even, cool room temperature – too cool and the ferment will take longer than you'd like, too warm and the sauerkraut may become mouldy or ferment too quickly, leading to a less than perfect result.

5 The cabbage will become increasingly sour the longer it's fermented, so taste it now and again. When you like the flavour, transfer it to smaller sterilised jars and keep it in the fridge for up to 6 months.

Nutrition: *per tbsp*
kcal 33 fat 0g saturates 0g carbs 5g sugars 5g fibre 3g protein 1g salt 2.1g

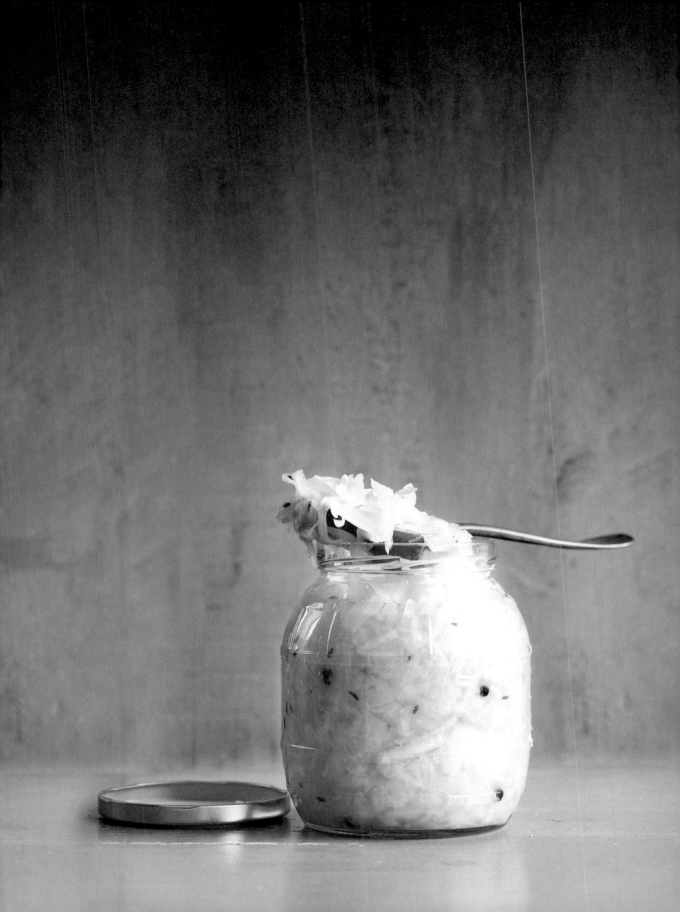

Quick kimchi

This Korean classic is made by fermenting cabbage and carrots in a tangy, spicy sauce – try this speedy version for a tasty side dish.

PREP 20 mins plus fermenting NO COOK 6–8

- 1 Chinese cabbage
- 3 garlic cloves, crushed
- 2.5cm piece ginger, grated
- 2 tbsp fish sauce (optional)
- 2 tbsp sriracha chilli sauce or chilli paste
- 1 tbsp golden caster sugar
- 3 tbsp rice vinegar
- 8 radishes, coarsely grated
- 2 carrots, cut into matchsticks or coarsely grated
- 4 spring onions, finely shredded

1 Slice the cabbage into 2.5cm strips. Tip into a bowl, mix with 1 tbsp sea salt, then set aside for 1 hr. Meanwhile, make the kimchi paste by blending the garlic, ginger, fish sauce (if using), chilli sauce, sugar and rice vinegar together in a small bowl.

2 Rinse the cabbage under cold running water, drain and dry thoroughly. Transfer to a large bowl and toss through the paste, along with the radishes, carrot and spring onions. Serve straight away or pack into a large jar, seal and leave to ferment at room temperature overnight, then chill. Will keep in the fridge for up to 2 weeks – the flavour will improve the longer it's left.

Nutrition: *per serving (8)*
kcal 42 fat 1g saturates 0g carbs 7g sugars 6g fibre 2g protein 1g salt 2g

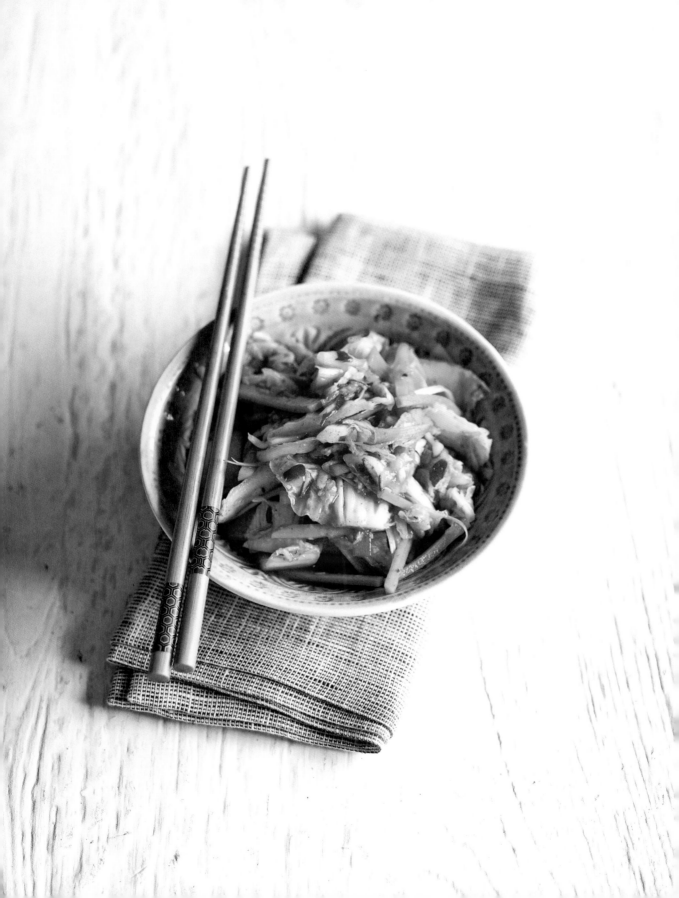

Avocado, labneh & roasted carrot salad

Labneh is made by straining yogurt until thick and creamy. It's also good spread on crackers or served with falafel.

PREP 20 mins plus straining COOK 30 mins 2

- 200g full-fat bio yogurt
- grated zest 1 lime, plus 1 tbsp juice, cut into wedges, to serve
- ½ small pack coriander leaves, finely chopped
- 300g carrots, cut into batons
- 1 tbsp extra virgin rapeseed oil
- ½ tsp ground cumin
- 1 ripe but firm avocado
- 50g bag mixed salad leaves
- 1 tbsp mixed seeds (such as sunflower, pumpkin, sesame and linseed)

1 To make the labneh, mix the yogurt, lime zest and coriander together in a bowl. Line another small bowl with a square of muslin. Spoon the yogurt mixture into the bowl, pull up the ends of the muslin and tie the yogurt into a ball. Tie the ends of the muslin onto a wooden spoon and suspend over a bowl or jug. Place in the fridge overnight to strain.

2 Heat oven to 200C/180C fan/gas 6. Toss the carrots with 1 tsp of the oil, 2 tsp of the lime juice, the cumin and lots of ground black pepper. Tip onto a foil-lined baking tray and roast for 20 mins. Turn the carrots and return to the oven for a further 10 mins or until tender and lightly browned. Set aside.

3 Cut the avocado in half and remove the stone. Scoop out the flesh from each half in one piece with a serving spoon. Slice on a chopping board, then toss with the remaining lime juice.

4 Untie the labneh and spread it over 2 plates, top with the salad leaves, carrots and avocado. Drizzle over the remaining oil, sprinkle with the seeds and serve with lime wedges.

Nutrition: *per serving*
kcal 370 fat 25g saturates 5g carbs 21g sugars 19g fibre 9g protein 9g salt 0.3g

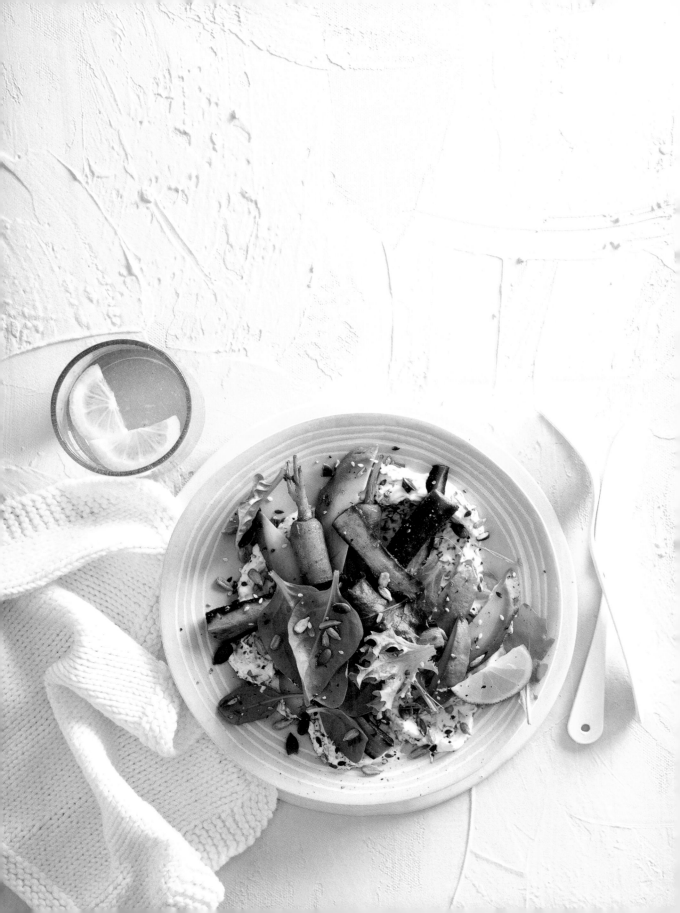

Nutty cinnamon & yogurt dipper

This speedy snack is great for hungry mouths after school.

🕐 PREP 5 mins NO COOK 🍽 1

- 100g natural Greek yogurt
- 1 tbsp nut butter (try almond or cashew)
- ¼ tsp ground cinnamon
- 1 tsp honey

TO SERVE
- Apple wedges (tossed in a little lemon juice to prevent them turning brown)
- celery sticks
- carrot sticks
- mini rice cakes or crackers (choose gluten-free brands if necessary)

In a small tub, mix together the yogurt, nut butter, cinnamon and honey. Serve with apple wedges (tossed in a little lemon juice to prevent them turning brown), celery or carrot sticks, and mini rice cakes or crackers.

Nutrition: *per serving*
kcal 250 fat 18g saturates 8g carbs 14g sugars 10g fibre 0g protein 8g salt 0.2g

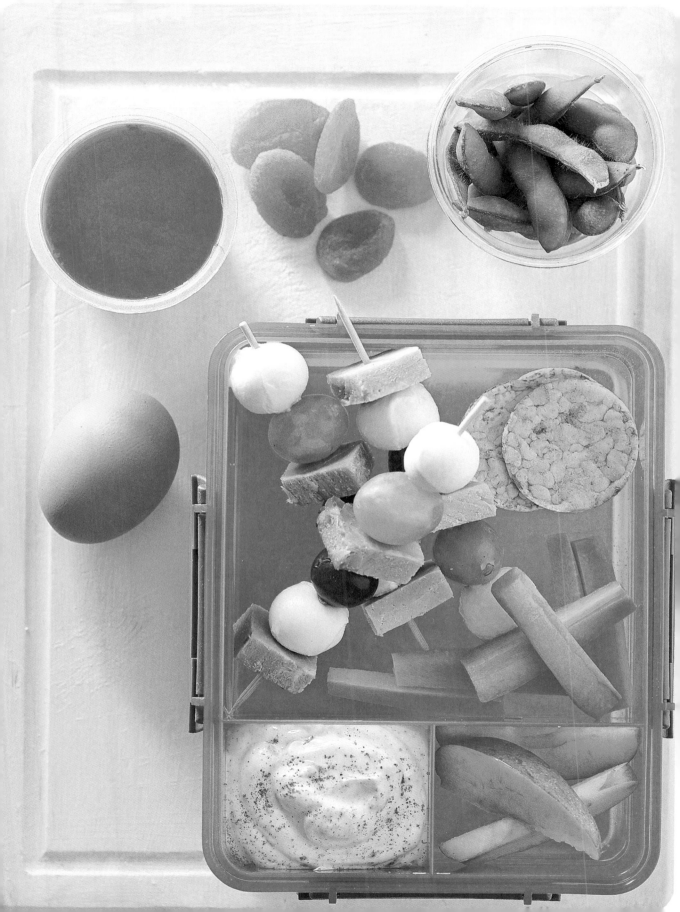

Smoked salmon, miso & sesame tartine

A smart starter or breakfast dish using fermented miso paste.

🕐 PREP 5 mins COOK 5 mins 🥧 2

- 2 tbsp white miso
- 2 tbsp tahini
- 4 slices sourdough bread
- 100g pack smoked salmon
- ½ cucumber, cut into thin rounds
- ½ tbsp black sesame seeds

Mix the miso with the tahini and 1 tbsp water in a bowl to make a spreadable paste. Toast the bread, then top with the miso paste, salmon, cucumber and black sesame seeds.

Nutrition: *per serving*
kcal 562 fat 21g saturates 3g carbs 59g sugars 4g fibre 5g protein 32g salt 3.7g

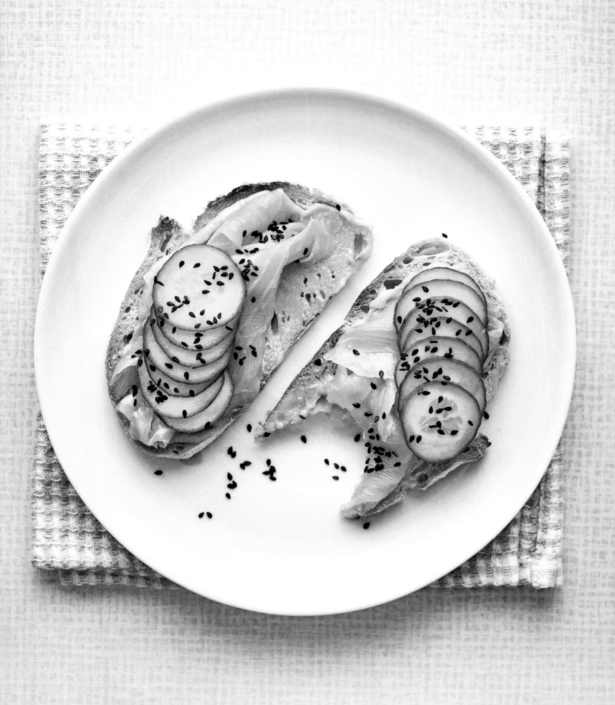

Sea veg & duck egg on sourdough

Sourdough bread is made with a fermented flour paste called a starter, instead of yeast. It's great for the gut and can be used in so many ways.

PREP 15 mins COOK 10 mins 2

- 50g sea purslane, samphire or sea kale, washed and trimmed of woody stalks
- 2 tbsp butter
- 150g mixed seasonal mushrooms, cleaned
- 2 tbsp extra virgin rapeseed oil
- 2 duck eggs
- 2 large slices sourdough
- 1 garlic clove, crushed
- squeeze of lemon

1 Bring a pan of water to the boil, add the sea vegetables and blanch for about 30 secs, then drain.
2 Melt half the butter in a frying pan, add the mushrooms and season. Fry for 8–10 mins or until golden-crusted and reduced in size. Meanwhile, heat the rapeseed oil in a frying pan and fry the eggs gently for a couple of mins. Toast the sourdough until golden. Transfer the sourdough to plates and keep warm.
3 Add the rest of the butter to the mushroom pan along with the garlic, cook for a further 1 min, then toss in the sea veg to warm through briefly. Season and add the lemon juice.
4 Top the sourdough with the eggs and scatter over the sea veg and mushrooms. Spoon over any butter from the pan and grind some seasoning over the yolks. Serve while hot.

Nutrition: *per serving*
kcal 495 fat 33g saturates 11g carbs 28g sugars 2g fibre 3g protein 19g salt 1.7g

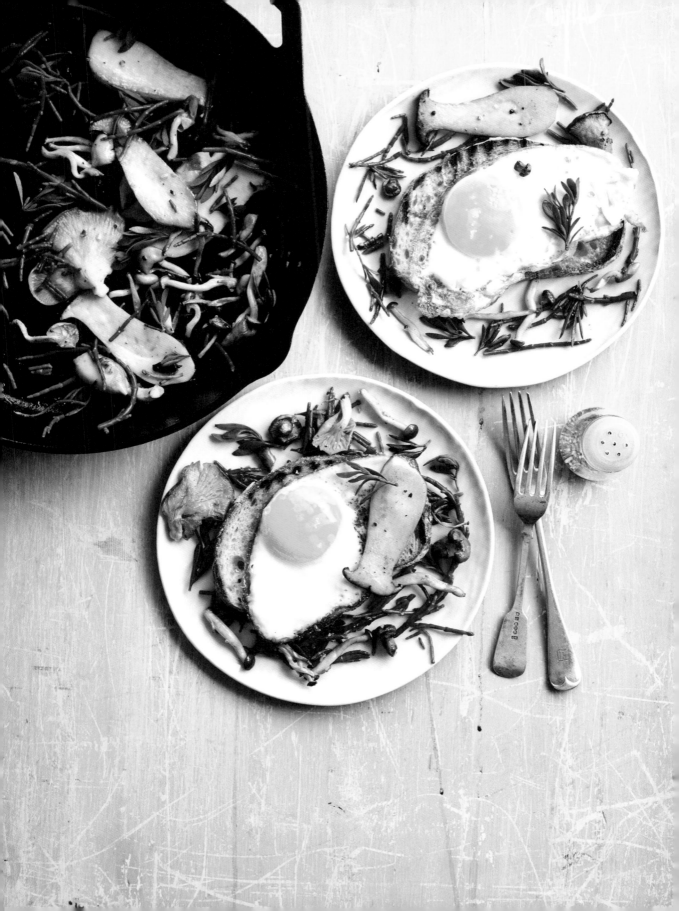

Miso aubergines

This vegan dish makes a simple and nutritious dinner. If you can't find wholemeal giant couscous, you could use bulghar wheat instead.

PREP 10 mins COOK 50 mins 2

- 2 small aubergines, halved
- vegetable oil, for roasting and frying
- 50g brown miso
- 100g giant couscous, wholemeal is nice
- 1 red chilli, thinly sliced
- ½ small pack coriander, leaves chopped

1 Heat oven to 180C/160C fan/ gas 4. With a sharp knife, criss-cross the flesh of the aubergines in a diagonal pattern, then place on a baking tray. Brush the flesh with 1 tbsp vegetable oil.

2 Mix the miso with 25ml water to make a thick paste. Spread the paste over the aubergines, then cover the tray with foil and roast in the centre of the oven for 30 mins.

3 Remove the foil and roast the aubergines for a further 15–20 mins, depending on their size, until tender.

4 Meanwhile, bring a saucepan of salted water to the boil and heat ½ tbsp vegetable oil over a medium-high heat in a frying pan. Add the couscous to the frying pan, toast for 2 mins until golden brown, then tip into the pan of boiling water and cook for 8–10 mins until tender (or following pack instructions). Drain well. Serve the aubergines with the couscous, topped with the chilli and a scattering of coriander leaves.

Nutrition: *per serving*
kcal 390 fat 12g saturates 1g carbs 51g sugars 8g fibre 11g protein 18g salt 2.3g

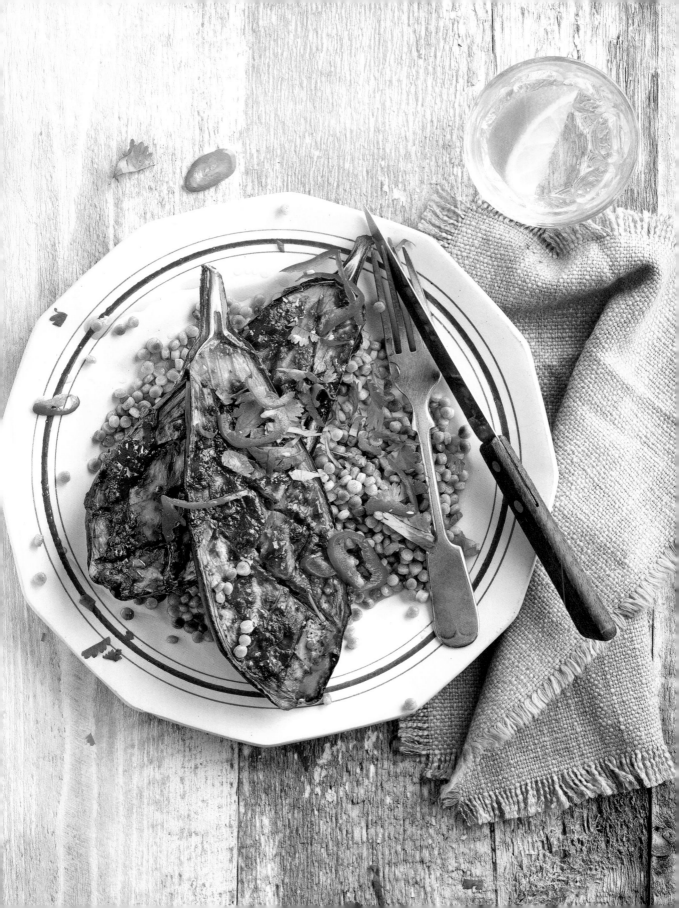

Chicken & chickpea salad with curry yogurt dressing

Use thick Greek, bio or natural yogurt when possible, its nutritional benefits are higher than that of low-fat yogurt.

🕐 PREP 15 mins COOK 15 mins 🥧 2

- 2 chicken breasts
- 200ml Greek yogurt
- 2 tsp mild curry powder
- juice ½ lemon
- small handful mint leaves, most chopped
- 400g can chickpeas, drained and rinsed
- 100g cherry tomatoes, quartered
- 1 small red onion, chopped
- 1 tbsp peanuts, crushed

1 Bring a pan of water to the boil. Add the chicken breasts and some salt, then put on the lid. Turn off the heat and leave for 15 mins until cooked through. Drain, then shred the chicken.
2 In a small bowl, mix the yogurt, curry powder, lemon juice, chopped mint and some seasoning.
3 Toss the chicken and chickpeas with half the dressing, and season. Arrange on 2 plates and scatter over the tomatoes, onion, remaining mint and peanuts. Drizzle any extra dressing over the top.

Nutrition: *per serving*
kcal 441 fat 18g saturates 8g carbs 21g sugars 8g fibre 7g protein 45g salt 1.2g

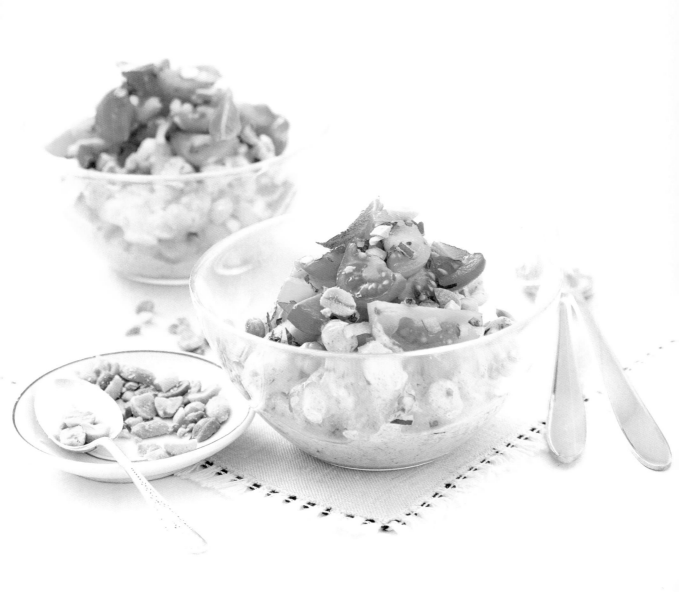

Salmon with miso vegetables

A Japanese-inspired meal with nutritious fish, broccoli and watercress served in a rich garlicky broth.

🕐 PREP 5 mins COOK 9 mins 🥧 2

- 8g pack instant miso soup
- 2 garlic cloves, finely grated
- 1 tbsp rice vinegar or white wine vinegar
- 100g thin-stemmed broccoli, cut into lengths and small florets
- 4 spring onions, chopped
- 100g beansprouts
- 2 big handfuls watercress (about 50-85g)
- 2 skinless salmon fillets

1 Make up the soup mix in a large pan with 500ml water and bring to the boil with the garlic and vinegar. Add the broccoli and spring onions, cover and cook for 5 mins.
2 Stir in the beansprouts and watercress, top with the salmon and cover again. Cook for 4 mins until the salmon flakes easily. Serve in bowls with a fork and spoon.

Nutrition: *per serving*
kcal 282 fat 15g saturates 3g carbs 6g sugars 4g fibre 5g protein 31g salt 1.2g

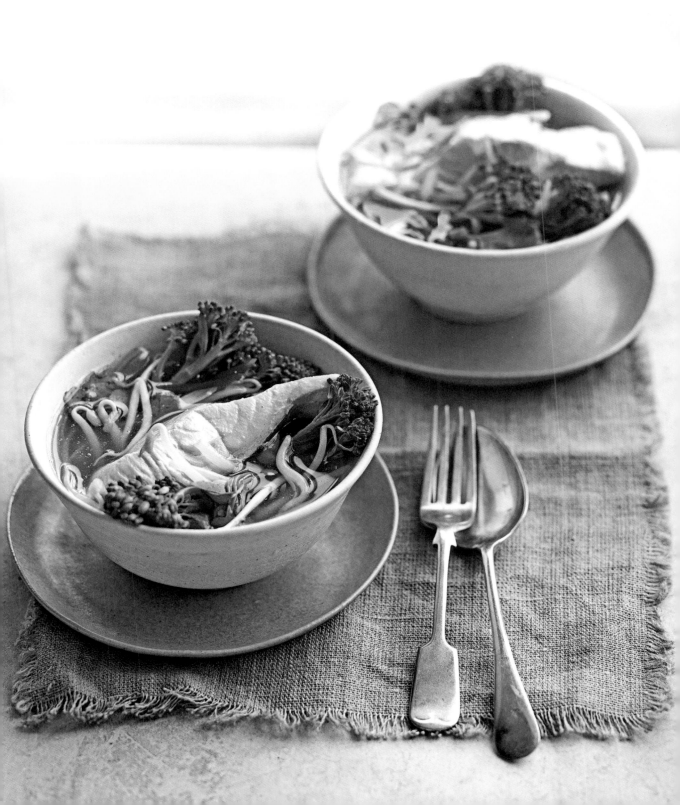

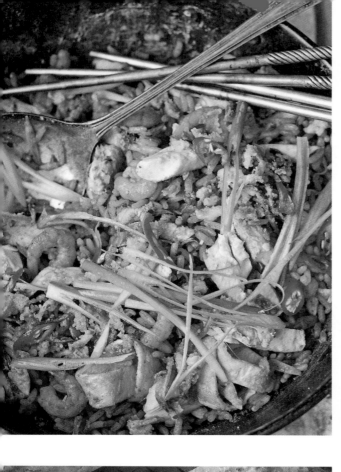
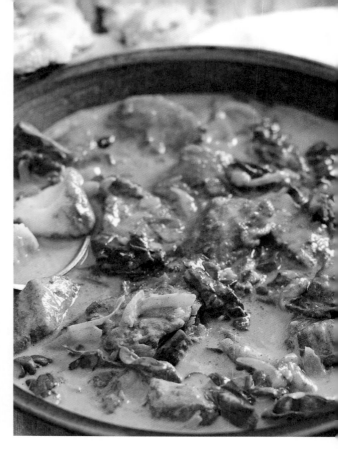
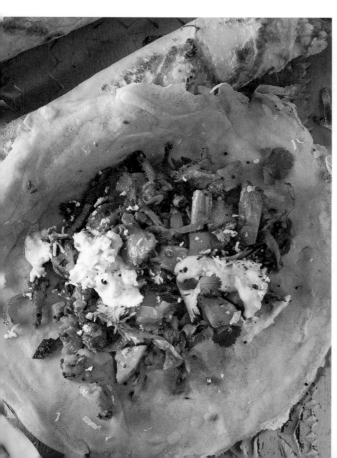
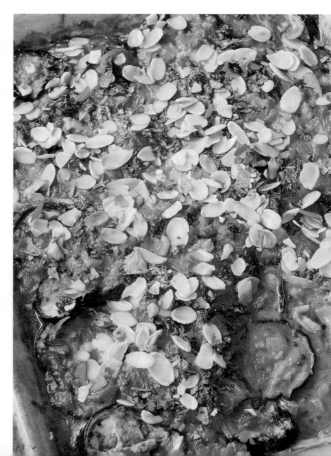

Chapter 8:

HERBS & SPICES

. . . .

Herbs and spices are wonderful little powerhouses of superfood goodness providing antioxidant, alkalizing and anti-inflammatory properties. Most are available in fresh or dried form – dried tend to be more intense in flavour, so go easy when adding for the first time. If you're using dried varieties, buy organic, where possible, so you optimize their goodness.

We've used basil and mint as a pesto to accompany our Roast leg of lamb (page 304) – basil is rich in heart-healthy nutrients and has anti-bacterial properties. Whilst mint, the classic partner to lamb, helps ease indigestion and bloating.

Using cinnamon in sweet recipes, like our Chai tea (page 294), is a smart way to help stabilize blood sugar spikes. That's because this delicious spice enhances the effect of insulin, which helps balance blood sugar. Another warm and aromatic spice, ginger, calms the digestive system and reduces inflammation, making it helpful for nausea, travel sickness, as well as painful joints and muscles. Along with garlic it has proven immune boosting properties. Other digestive settlers include aniseed, cardamom and fennel seeds.

One spice that has long held superfood status is turmeric. Its yellow pigments have powerful anti-inflammatory properties, which are said to rival that of ibuprofen. Like garlic, turmeric makes a great liver tonic – it enhances the flow of bile, which keeps the liver healthy. Use turmeric to alleviate joint pain, ease the effects of skin complaints like acne and eczema and even protect against cognitive decline.

Nasi goreng with sardines

You could also use mackerel or anchovies in this spicy rice dish.

PREP 20 mins COOK 20 mins 4

- 4 sardines, gutted
- 2 tbsp sunflower oil
- 2 eggs, beaten
- 6 spring onions, 4 chopped, 2 shredded
- 2 garlic cloves, crushed
- 1 tbsp shrimp paste
- ½ tsp turmeric
- 2 tsp tomato purée
- 2 red chillies, sliced
- 400g cooked rice (250g uncooked)
- 85g small prawns
- 1 tbsp soy sauce, plus extra to serve (optional)
- large handful coriander leaves
- 3 tbsp crispy shallot flakes (optional)
- finely sliced cucumber, to serve

1 Heat the grill to high and brush the sardines with a little oil. Grill for about 4 mins on each side until lightly blistered and cooked through, then set aside.

2 Heat half the remaining oil in a wok and cook the eggs to a thin omelette. Tip onto a plate to cool. Heat the rest of the oil in the same wok. Add the chopped spring onions, the garlic, shrimp paste, turmeric, tomato purée and half the chilli. Sizzle everything together to form a paste, then add the rice and prawns. Season with soy sauce and stir-fry for 5 mins until everything is combined and hot.

3 Roll up the omelette and finely shred. Flake the fish into large boneless chunks. Stir the omelette ribbons and fish into the rice, then scatter over the shredded spring onions, remaining chilli, coriander leaves and crispy shallot flakes (if using). Serve the rice with extra soy, if you like, and finely sliced cucumber on the side.

Nutrition: *per serving*
kcal 446 fat 20g saturates 5g carbs 30g sugars 1g fibre 0g protein 36g salt 2g

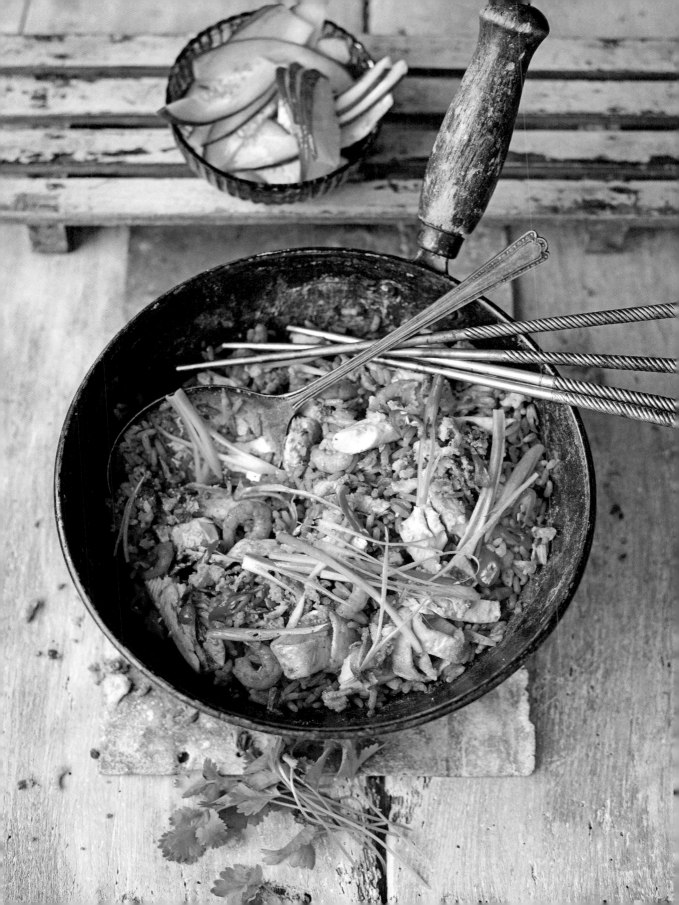

Cod & spinach yellow curry

This vibrant curry gets its gorgeous yellow colour from turmeric, a spice powerhouse, rich in the antioxidant curcumin.

PREP 10 mins COOK 20 mins | 2

- 1 tsp garam masala
- 1 tsp turmeric
- 1 tsp smoked paprika
- 250g cod fillet, cut into bite-sized chunks
- 2 tbsp groundnut oil (or any flavourless oil)
- 1 onion, finely sliced
- 2 garlic cloves, finely sliced
- thumb-sized piece ginger, peeled and grated
- 400g can coconut milk
- 100g fresh spinach
- cooked basmati rice and naan bread, to serve (optional)

1 In a small bowl, combine the spices. Coat the fish with half the spice mixture and some seasoning. Set aside.
   In a medium lidded frying pan, heat the oil over a medium heat. Add the onion, garlic and ginger, and fry for 8 mins until softened. Add the remaining spice mix and gently cook for 1 min to release the flavour of the spices.

2 Pour in the coconut milk, bring to the boil and simmer for 3–5 mins to reduce slightly, then add the cod and spinach. Pop the lid on and continue to cook for 5 mins or so until the spinach has wilted and the cod is cooked through. Season to taste and serve with basmati rice and naan bread, if you like.

Nutrition: *per serving*
kcal 651 fat 49g saturates 32g carbs 23g sugars 9g fibre 3g protein 29g salt 0.5g

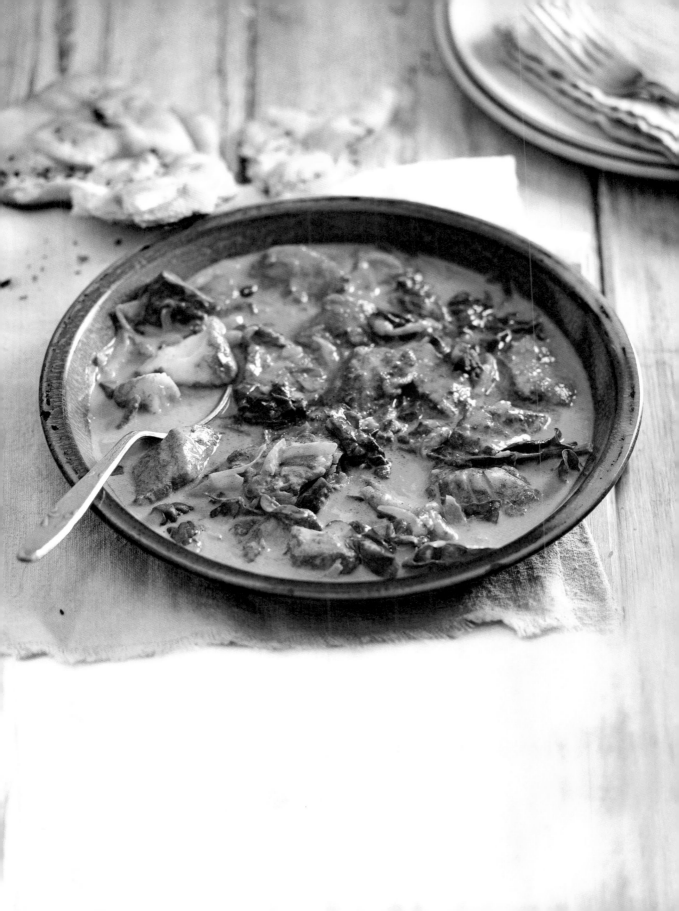

Chai tea

Sweet and spicy chai tea makes a delicious alternative to your regular brew.

PREP 2 mins COOK 15 mins 2

- 2 mugs milk (or use almond milk)
- 2 English Breakfast tea bags
- 6 cracked cardamom pods
- ½ cinnamon stick
- a grating of fresh nutmeg
- 2 cloves
- 2–4 tsp light brown soft sugar

1 Heat the milk in a saucepan over a very low heat. Empty the contents of the tea bags into the pan, then add the cracked cardamom pods, cinnamon stick, nutmeg and cloves.
2 Sweeten with light brown soft sugar to taste (chai tea should be sweet, but use less if you like), then leave to infuse, but not boil, for 10 mins. Strain into mugs and enjoy.

Nutrition: *per cup*
kcal 100 fat 3g saturates 2g carbs 13g sugars 11g fibre 0g protein 5g salt 0.2g

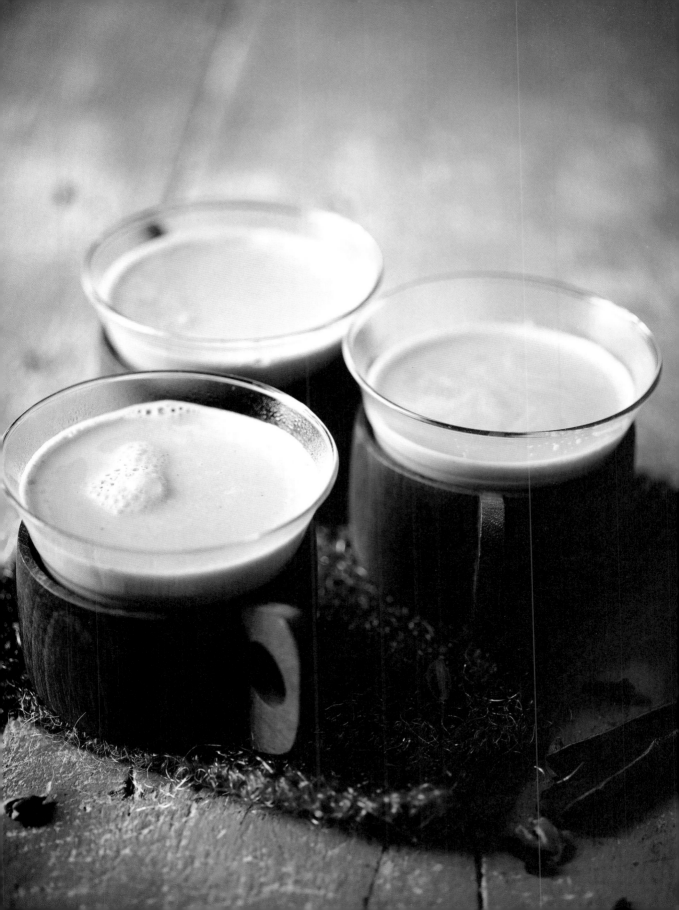

Sweet potato masala dosa

Dosas are a popular Indian pancake, often filled with spiced mashed potato.

PREP 40 mins COOK 50 mins 4

FOR THE DOSA
- 100g gram flour
- 100g plain flour
- 200ml milk

FOR THE MASALA FILLING
- 4 sweet potatoes (about 750g/1lb 10oz), peeled and chopped into small cubes
- 3 tbsp vegetable or sunflower oil
- 2 tsp black mustard seeds
- 2 tsp fennel seeds
- 2 tsp cumin seeds
- 1 fat red chilli, chopped (deseeded if you don't like it too hot)
- 1 large onion, halved and thinly sliced
- 4 garlic cloves, crushed
- thumb-sized piece ginger, peeled and finely chopped
- small bunch coriander, stalks only, finely chopped (save the leaves for the raita)
- 2 tbsp fresh or dried curry leaves
- 1 tsp ground turmeric
- 1 tsp ground coriander
- Indian chutneys, raita and pickles to serve
- zest 1 lime, juice of ½, the other ½ cut into wedges to serve

1. Measure the flours into a bowl, add the milk, season and add 300ml water. Whisk to a smooth batter, cover with cling film and chill for 24 hrs or up to 5 days.
2. Heat oven to 200C/180C fan/gas 6. Toss the sweet potato in a drizzle of the oil and spread out on a large baking tray. Cook for 20 mins, until soft and starting to caramelise. Meanwhile, heat the remaining oil in a pan and fry the mustard, fennel and cumin seeds for 30 secs or so until fragrant. Stir in the chilli, onion, garlic, ginger, coriander stalks and curry leaves, and cook over a low heat for 10 mins until the onion is soft. Stir in the ground spices, then add 100ml water and bubble to bring all the flavours together.
3. Stir the sweet potato into the pan and season well. Use the back of your spoon to crush some of the sweet potato, leaving some pieces chunkier – the mixture should resemble very chunky mash. Keep the mixture warm until the pancakes are ready (or leave it to cool, then chill for up to 2 days – gently reheat in the pan or microwave before continuing).
4. Heat the oven to its lowest setting and put a plate inside ready to keep the dosas warm. If the dosa batter has thickened in the fridge, thin it with a splash of water – it should be the consistency of double cream. Use a little oil to grease a large frying or crêpe pan, wiping out the excess oil with some kitchen paper. Pour a ladleful of batter into the centre of the pan and quickly swirl it around to fill the surface, getting the pancakes as thin as you can. When the surface of the pancake looks almost dry, spoon a quarter of the filling down the centre. When the pancake is deep golden-brown and crisp on the underside, roll it up in the pan to encase the filling, cook for 1 min more, then transfer to the oven to keep warm while you continue cooking the remaining dosas.
5. Serve the dosas with raita, lime wedges and remaining coriander leaves, with your favourite Indian chutneys and pickles on the side.

Nutrition: *per serving*
kcal 803 fat 36g saturates 22g carbs 96g sugars 35g fibre 18g protein 16g salt 0.4g

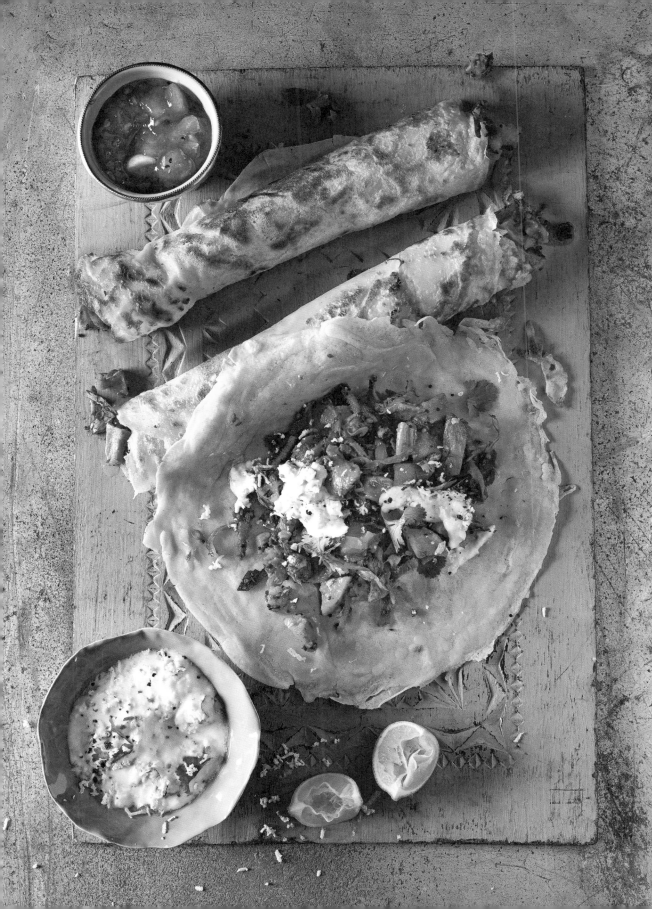

Spiced aubergine bake

This is vegan comfort food at its best – layer up slices of aubergine with a spicy coconut milk and tomato sauce for a hearty, warming meal.

PREP 15 mins COOK 1 hour 4-6

- 4 aubergines, cut into 5mm-1cm slices
- 3 tbsp vegetable oil
- 2 tbsp coconut oil
- 2 large onions, chopped
- 3 garlic cloves, crushed
- 1 tbsp black mustard seeds
- ½ tbsp fenugreek seeds
- 1 tbsp garam masala
- ¼ tsp hot chilli powder
- 1 cinnamon stick
- 1 tsp ground cumin
- 1 tsp ground coriander
- 2 x 400g cans chopped tomatoes
- 200ml coconut milk
- sugar, to taste
- 2 tbsp flaked almonds
- small bunch coriander, roughly chopped (optional)

1 Heat oven to 220C/200C fan/gas 7. Generously brush each aubergine slice with vegetable oil and place in a single layer on a baking tray, or two if they don't fit on one. Cook on the low shelves for 10 mins, then turn over and cook for a further 5–10 mins until they are golden. Reduce the oven to 180C/160C fan/gas 4.

2 Heat the coconut oil in a large, heavy-based frying pan and add the onions. Cover and sweat on a low heat for about 5 mins until softened. Add the garlic, mustard seeds, fenugreek seeds, garam masala, chilli powder, cinnamon stick, cumin and ground coriander. Cook for a few secs until it starts to smell beautiful and aromatic.

3 Pour the chopped tomatoes and coconut milk into the spiced onions and stir well. Check the seasoning and add a little sugar, salt or pepper to taste.

4 Spoon a third of the tomato sauce on the bottom of a 2-litre ovenproof dish. Layer with half the aubergine slices. Spoon over a further third of tomato sauce, then the remaining aubergine slices, and finish with the rest of the sauce. Sprinkle over the flaked almonds and coriander (if using), reserving some to serve, and bake for 25–30 mins. Serve garnished with more coriander.

Nutrition: *per serving (6)*
kcal 318 fat 20g saturates 9g carbs 19g sugars 15g fibre 12g protein 8g salt 0.2g

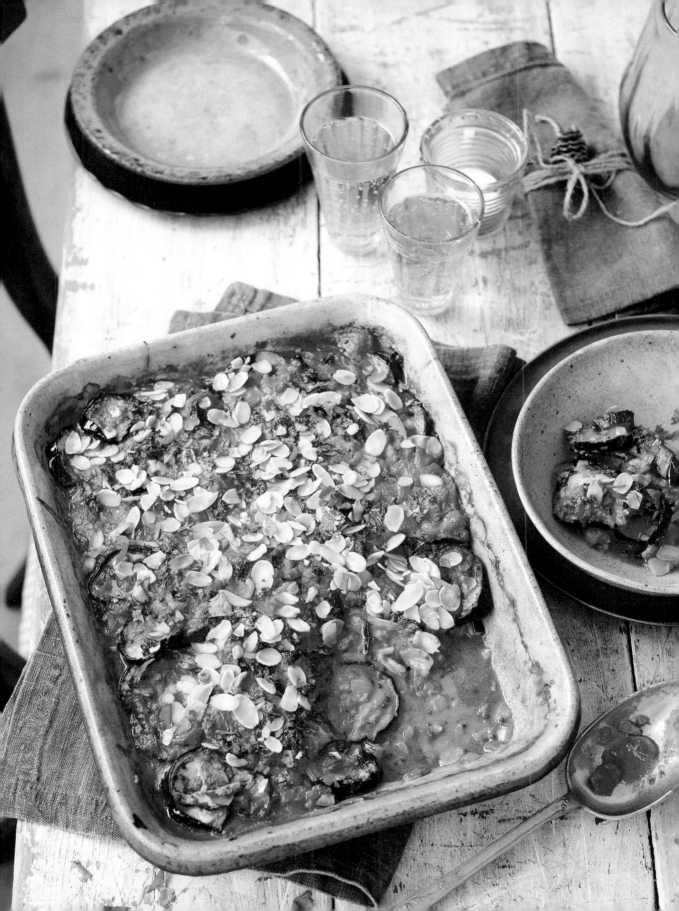

Tamarind aubergine with black rice, mint & feta

Fresh herbs add vibrant flavours and pack in the nutrients in this exciting dish.

🕐 PREP 25 mins COOK 40 mins 🍽 4

- 2 large aubergines
- 4 tsp tamarind paste
- 2 tsp sesame oil
- 1 red chilli, deseeded and thinly sliced
- 1 tbsp sesame seeds
- 200g black rice
- 6 spring onions, finely sliced
- 100g feta, crumbled
- 2 small packs mint, roughly chopped
- small pack coriander, roughly chopped, reserving a few leaves, to serve
- zest 1 large lime

FOR THE DRESSING
- 2 tbsp dark soy sauce
- juice 1 lime
- 5cm piece ginger, peeled and finely grated (juices and all)
- pinch of sugar

1 Heat oven to 200C/180C fan/gas 6. Cut the aubergines in half lengthways and, with the tip of a knife, score the flesh deeply in a criss-cross diamond pattern – but don't pierce the skin. Press on the edges of the halves to open the cuts. In a small bowl, combine the tamarind paste and sesame oil. Brush the mixture over the aubergine, pushing it into the cuts. Place on a baking tray, sprinkle over the chilli and sesame seeds, then roast, cut-side up, for 25–35 mins or until the flesh is really soft.

2 Put the rice in a small sieve and wash under running water for 1 min until the water runs clear. Tip the rice into a small saucepan and add 650ml cold water. Bring to the boil, reduce the heat and simmer for about 35 mins until the rice is tender. Drain under cold running water.

3 Make the dressing by whisking all the ingredients together with a pinch of salt. Adjust the seasoning to taste, adding a little more sugar, salt or lime juice, if you like.

4 In a big bowl, mix together the black rice, spring onions, feta, mint, chopped coriander, and the lime zest and dressing. Sprinkle the reserved coriander leaves over the aubergine halves and serve with the rice.

Nutrition: *per serving*
kcal 355 fat 10g saturates 4g carbs 46g sugars 11g fibre 11g protein 16g salt 2.3g

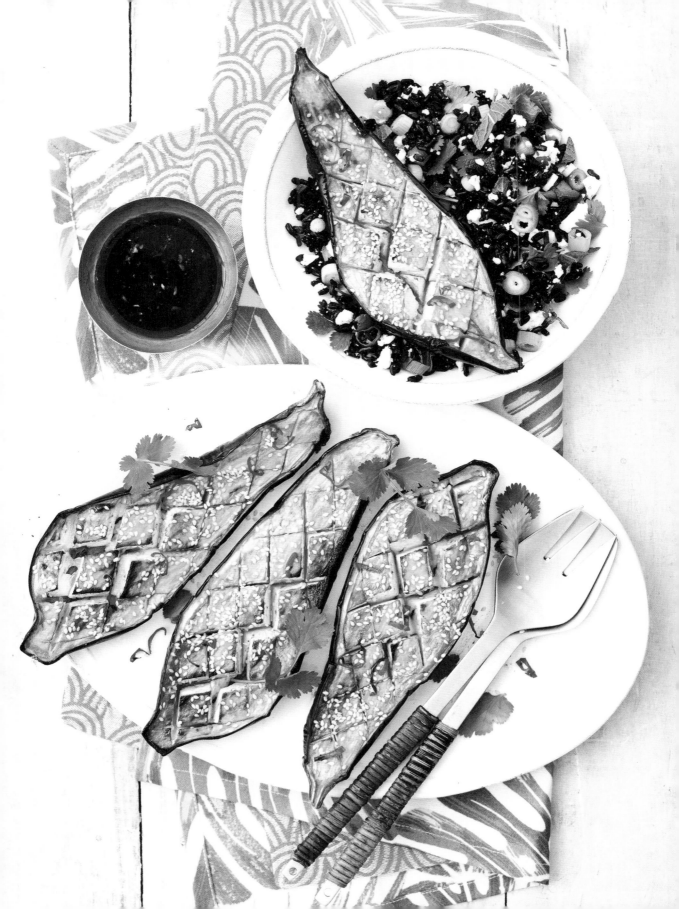

Tumeric smoothie bowl

Full of warming and nourishing ingredients, this creamy breakfast bowl can be ready in just 10 minutes.

PREP 10 mins NO COOK 2

- 10cm fresh turmeric, or 2 tsp ground turmeric
- 3 tbsp coconut milk yogurt or the cream skimmed from the top of canned coconut milk
- 50g gluten-free oats
- 1 tbsp cashew butter (or a handful cashews)
- 2 bananas, peeled and roughly chopped
- ½ tsp ground cinnamon
- 1 tbsp chia seeds or chopped nuts, to serve

Peel the turmeric root, if using, and grate. Put all ingredients in a blender with 600ml water and blend until smooth. Serve in a bowl with chia seeds or some chopped nuts sprinkled over.

Nutrition: *per serving*
kcal 291 fat 10g saturates 4g carbs 40g sugars 20g fibre 5g protein 7g salt 0g

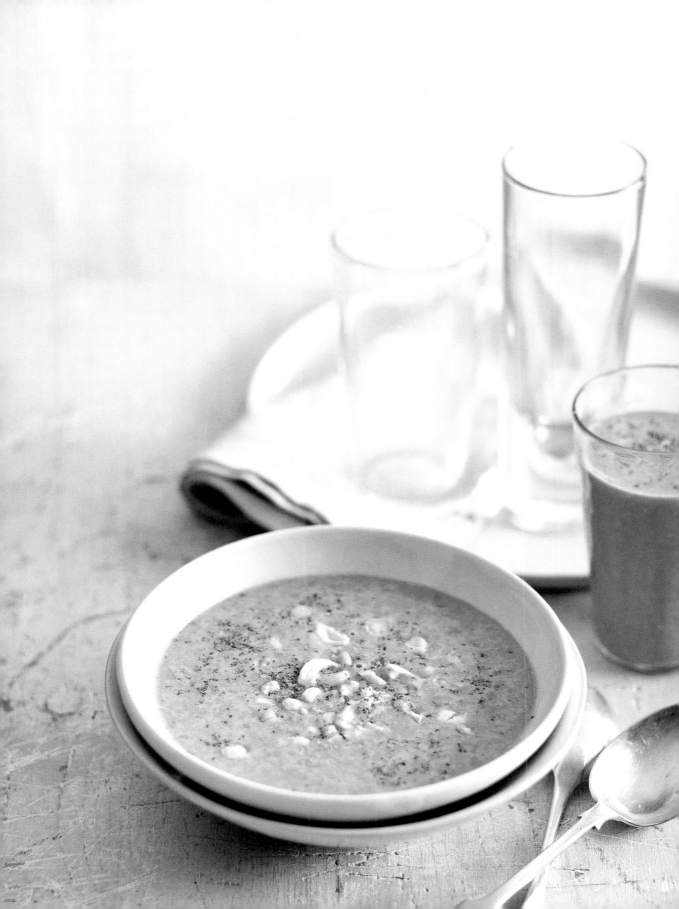

Moroccan harira

This is a healthy vegetarian version of the classic Moroccan soup with plenty of cumin, turmeric and cinnamon, each offering different health benefits, plus it's low in fat and calories too.

🕐 PREP 15 mins COOK 40 mins 🥧 4

- 1–2 tbsp extra virgin rapeseed oil
- 2 large onions, finely chopped
- 4 garlic cloves, chopped
- 2 tsp turmeric
- 2 tsp cumin
- ½ tsp cinnamon
- 2 red chillies, deseeded and sliced
- 500g carton passata
- 1.7 litres reduced-salt vegetable bouillon
- 175g dried green lentils
- 2 carrots, chopped into small pieces
- 1 sweet potato, peeled and diced
- 5 celery sticks, chopped into small pieces
- ⅔ small pack coriander, few sprigs reserved, the rest chopped
- 1 lemon, cut into 4 wedges, to serve

1 Heat the oil in a large non-stick sauté pan over a medium heat and fry the onions and garlic until starting to soften. Tip in the spices and chilli, stir briefly, then pour in the passata and stock. Add the lentils, carrots, sweet potato and celery, and bring to the boil.

2 Cover the pan and leave to simmer for 30 mins, then cook uncovered for a further 5–10 mins until the vegetables and lentils are tender. Stir in the chopped coriander and serve in bowls with lemon wedges for squeezing over, and the reserved coriander sprinkled over.

Nutrition: *per serving*
kcal 335 fat 6g saturates 1g carbs 48g sugars 21g fibre 13g protein 16g salt 0.2g

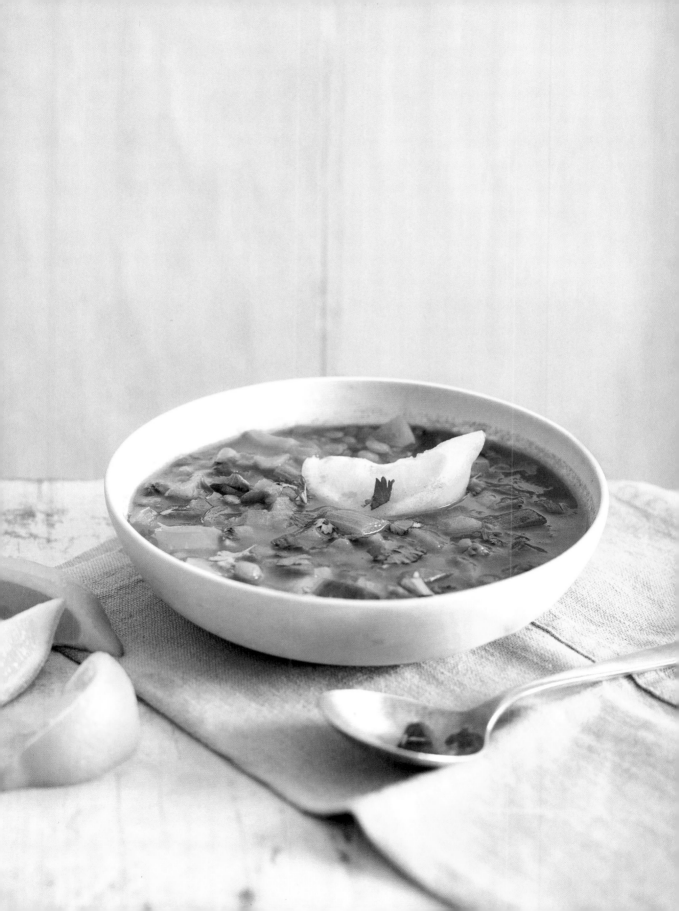

Roast leg of lamb with basil & mint pesto

Add a fresh twist to your usual Sunday lunch with a fragrant pesto.

🕐 PREP 15 mins COOK 1 hr 45 mins 🕐 6

- 2kg lamb leg, skin scored
- fresh garden herbs, to serve (optional)
- sliced lemon, to serve (optional)

FOR THE PESTO
- 1 small garlic clove, roughly chopped
- small pack basil, leaves only
- small pack mint, leaves only
- 25g pine nuts
- 25g grated Parmesan
- 125ml extra virgin olive oil
- juice ½ lemon

1 First, make the pesto. Put all the ingredients (except the olive oil and lemon juice) and a pinch of salt into the small bowl of a food processor. Pulse until very finely chopped. While the processor is on, drizzle the olive oil in to make a paste. Tip the pesto into a small bowl and stir in the lemon juice.

2 Heat oven to 200C/180C fan/gas 6. Put the scored lamb leg in a large roasting tin and use half the pesto to generously coat the skin and flesh, pressing it between all the cracks for extra juiciness. Put the rest of the pesto in the fridge, covered with cling film, and remove just before serving.

3 Roast the lamb for 1 hr 45 mins. Check during cooking that it's not drying out – if the base of the roasting tin starts to look dry, spread a little more pesto over the top of the lamb.

4 Remove the lamb from the tin, cover with foil and leave to rest for 30–40 mins before serving on lemon slices and fresh garden herbs, if you like. Carve at the table and serve with the remaining pesto to drizzle over.

Nutrition: *per serving*
kcal 644 fat 49g saturates 15g carbs 1g sugars 0g fibre 0g protein 51g salt 0.4g

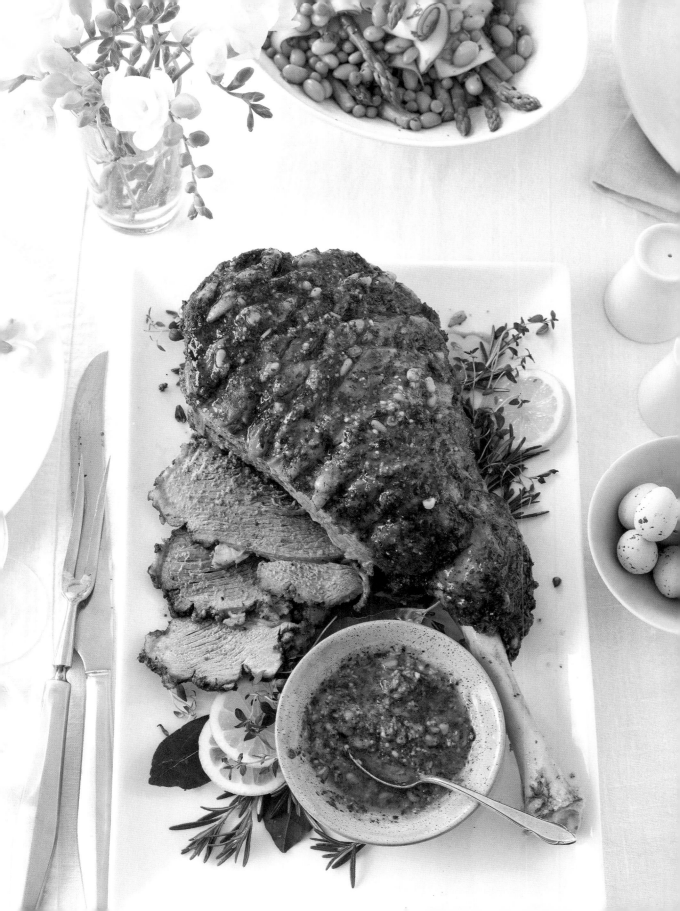

Spiced turkey patties with fruity quinoa salad

Spice up lean meatballs with coriander and cumin seeds, then serve on a salad of quinoa, red onions, carrots, pomegranate and parsley.

PREP 20 mins COOK 40 mins 4

- 4 carrots, peeled and cut into thin batons
- 3 red onions, 2½ cut into chunky wedges (roots intact) and ½ grated
- 2 tbsp olive oil
- 200g quinoa
- 2 tsp coriander seeds
- 2 tsp cumin seeds
- 400g turkey mince
- 25g fresh wholemeal breadcrumbs
- 3 garlic cloves, crushed
- 4 tbsp full-fat Greek yogurt
- few dashes of Tabasco sauce
- 1 pomegranate, deseeded over a bowl to catch the juices
- 2 oranges, segmented
- large pack parsley, roughly chopped

1 Heat oven to 220C/200C fan/gas 7. Tip the carrots and onion wedges into a roasting tin. Toss in 1 tbsp olive oil, season and roast, stirring once, for 30 mins or so until tender.

2 Meanwhile, cook the quinoa following pack instructions, drain and put to one side. Heat a large, non-stick frying pan and toast the seeds for 1–2 mins until aromatic. Pop into a pestle and mortar and grind before tipping into a large bowl. Add the turkey, grated onion, breadcrumbs, most of the garlic and seasoning, then mix. Shape into 12 small patties. Heat the remaining oil in the same pan and fry the patties for 3–4 mins on each side until browned and cooked through.

3 In a small bowl, mix the yogurt, remaining garlic, Tabasco, 1 tbsp of water and seasoning. Toss together the drained quinoa, pomegranate seeds and juice, orange segments, parsley and roasted veg and some seasoning. Serve with the patties and spiced yogurt.

Nutrition: *per serving*
kcal 526 fat 15g saturates 5g carbs 54g sugars 25g fibre 12g protein 37g salt 0.4g

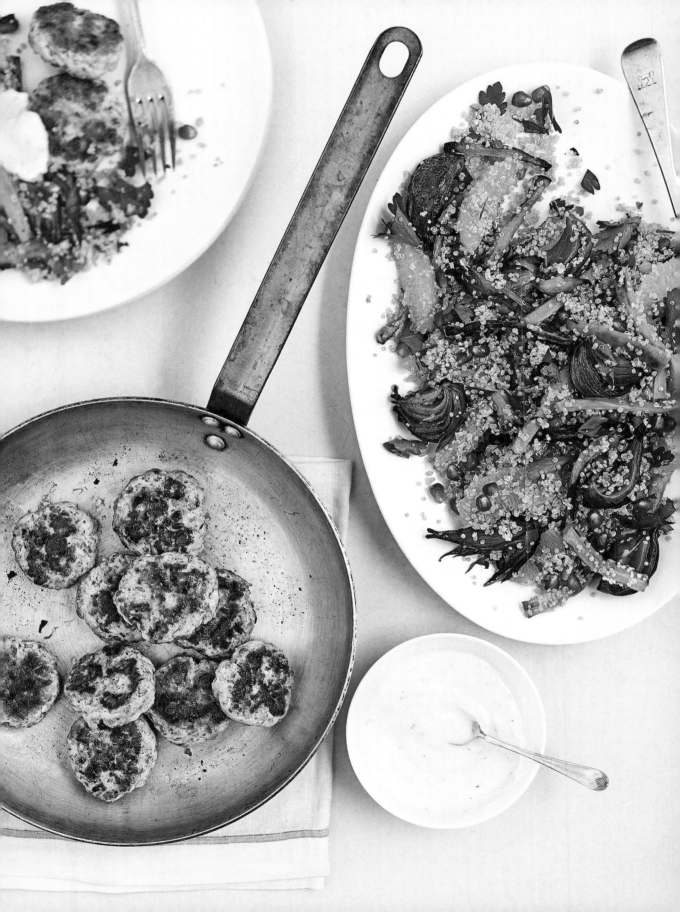

Winter veg curry with fruity raita

Use hardy root veg in this Asian-inspired spice pot. We used pumpkin, carrots and parsnips, teamed with tomatoes.

PREP 20 mins COOK 1 hr 4

- 2 tbsp vegetable oil
- 2 onions, thinly sliced
- ½ pumpkin, winter squash or butternut squash, cut into cubes
- 4 carrots, cut into batons
- 2 parsnips, cut into batons
- 3 tbsp curry paste
- 8 large ripe tomatos, 2 cut into wedges
- 6 garlic cloves, peeled
- thumb-sized piece ginger, peeled and chopped
- small pack coriander, chopped
- 200g brown basmati rice
- 6 tbsp natural yogurt
- 100g mango, cut into cubes
- 1 tbsp mango chutney
- small pack toasted flaked almond

1 Heat the oil in a large lidded pan. Tip in the onions and cook for 10 mins until soft. Stir in the pumpkin, carrots and parsnips, and cook for 5 mins until they begin to soften. Add the curry paste and cook for another 3 mins.

2 In a bowl, whizz together the whole tomatoes, garlic and ginger until smooth, then pour over the vegetables, adding 200ml water. Save a handful of coriander to serve, and stir in the rest. Pop on the lid and simmer for 40 mins or until the vegetables are tender. Uncover, stir through the tomato wedges and reduce to thicken the sauce.

3 Meanwhile, cook the rice following pack instructions. Mix the yogurt, mango and chutney in a small bowl. Fork the rice into a serving dish and scatter the curry with remaining coriander and the almonds. Season, then serve alongside the rice and fruity yogurt.

Nutrition: *per serving*
kcal 511 fat 14g saturates 3g carbs 73g sugars 34g fibre 14g protein 14g salt 0.8g

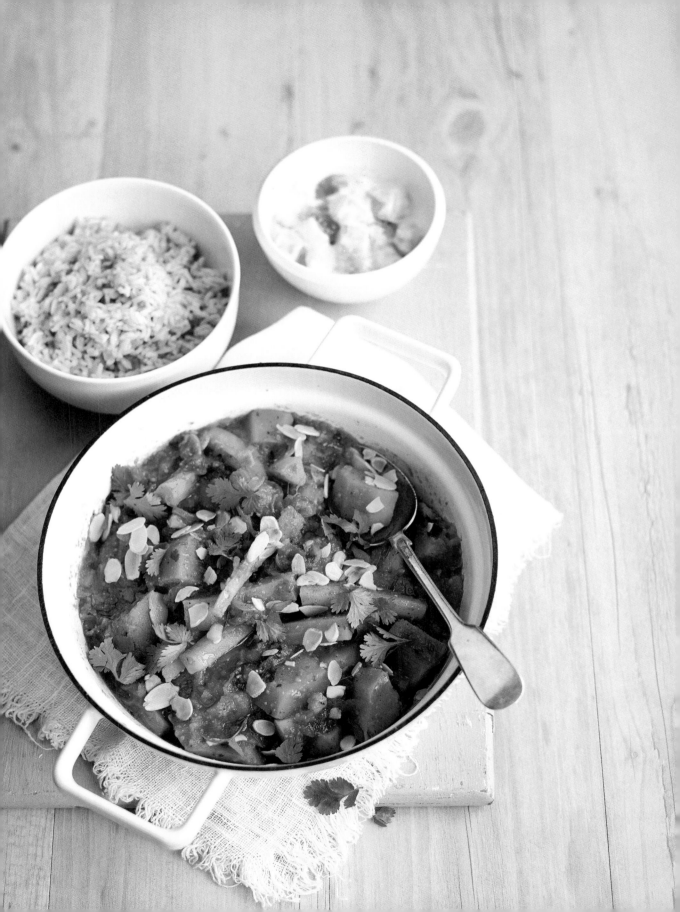

Indian oven chips

Spice up potato wedges with turmeric, ginger, garlic and fennel seeds for an Indian-inspired side dish – perfect to share with friends.

PREP 10 mins plus chilling COOK 55 mins 8

- 1kg floury potatoes such as Maris Piper, peeled and cut into chunky chips
- ½ tsp turmeric
- 3 tbsp sunflower oil
- thumb-sized piece ginger, peeled and chopped, or finely grated into a paste
- 3 garlic cloves, chopped or finely grated into a paste
- 1 tsp fennel seeds
- generous pinch of cayenne pepper

1 The day before you plan to eat them, tip the potatoes into a pan of cold water and add the turmeric and pinch of salt. Bring to the boil, and simmer gently for 2–3 mins until just cooked. Drain, leave to cool, then chill overnight if you can.

2 Heat oven to 200C/180C fan/gas 6. Drizzle 1 tbsp of the oil in a shallow roasting tin (preferably non-stick), and place in the oven. Pour the rest of the oil into a large bowl and add the ginger, garlic, fennel seeds and cayenne pepper. Tip the cold chips into the bowl and gently toss with your fingers until evenly coated. Remove the tray from the oven and scatter over the chips. Use a spatula to coat the chips in the hot oil, then lay them out in a single layer and roast for 30 mins. Use the spatula to turn, then return to the oven for 15 mins until crisp and golden.

Nutrition: *per serving*
kcal 140 fat 4g saturates 1g carbs 21g sugars 1g fibre 2g protein 3g salt 0g

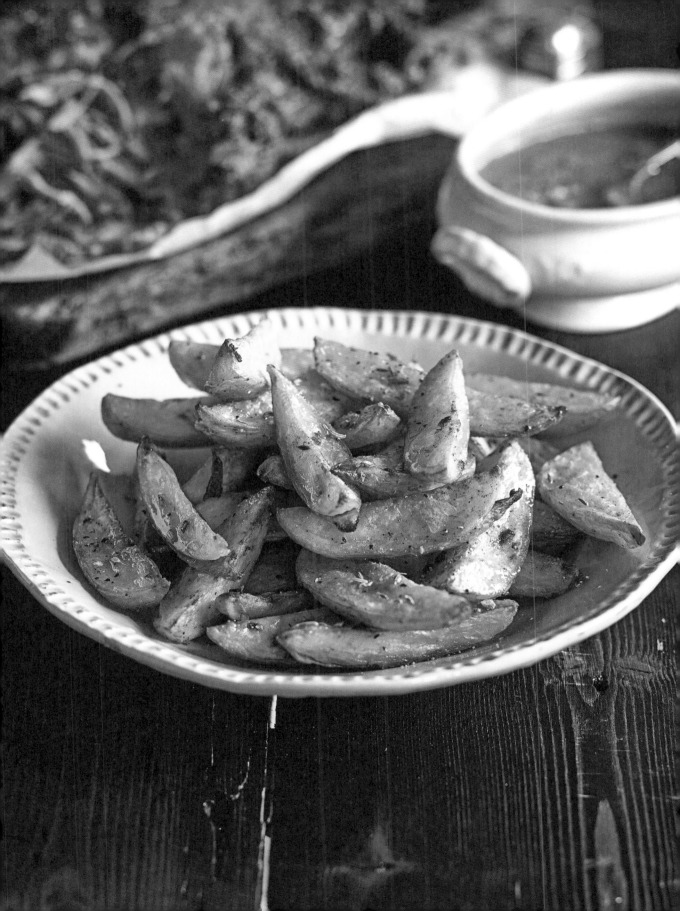

Lentil & bacon soup

Blend your storecupboard pulses with cumin, turmeric and garlic to create this robust soup with crispy pancetta topping.

⏱ PREP 5 mins COOK 35 mins 🍽 3

- 1 tbsp olive oil
- 1 onion, diced
- 2 x 70g packs pancetta cubes
- 1 carrot (about 120g), finely diced
- 1 tsp ground cumin
- ½ tsp turmeric
- 2 garlic cloves, finely chopped
- 1 chilli, sliced
- 2 low-salt stock cubes
- 250g red lentils, rinsed

1 Heat the olive oil in a large saucepan. Add the onion, 1 pack of pancetta and the carrot. Cook on a low-medium heat for 10 minutes until the onions are soft.
2 Add the cumin, turmeric, garlic and chilli and cook for a further 1—2 minutes until the aromas are released.
3 Pour in 1.25 litres of boiling water, crumble in the stock cubes and add the lentils. Bring to a simmer and cook for 20 mins, stirring occasionally to ensure the lentils aren't sticking.
4 Meanwhile, fry the remaining lardons in a small frying pan for about 10 minutes until crispy. You don't need to add any oil as plenty will run from the Serve the pancetta sprinkled over the soup.

Nutrition: *per serving*
kcal 493 fat 19.1g saturates 6.6g carbs 50.6g sugars 7.3g fibre 7.7g protein 29.5g salt 1.6g

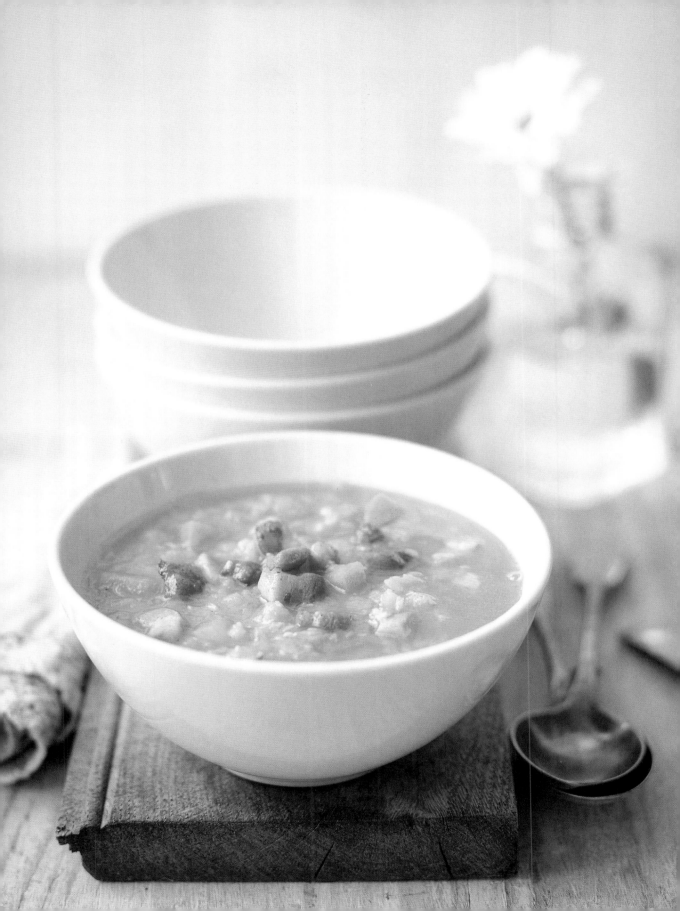

Curried haddock kedgeree

A classic kedgeree designed to fill you with warmth and spice. This gluten-free family meal is an easy midweek fix.

PREP 10 mins COOK 15 mins 4

- 500ml double cream
- thumb-sized piece ginger, peeled and grated
- ½ tsp turmeric
- 2 tsp ground cumin
- 2 tsp garam masala
- 400g undyed smoked haddock fillets (skin on)
- 300g cooked brown basmati rice
- 200g frozen peas
- 2 large eggs, boiled for 7 mins, peeled and cut into quarters
- 1 small pack coriander, leaves roughly chopped

1 Pour the cream into a large sauté pan with a lid. Stir in the ginger and spices, then submerge the smoked haddock fillets, skin-side up. Put the lid on, bring the cream slowly to the boil, then remove from the heat and leave to cool. Flake the fish into a bowl in large pieces, discarding the skin.

2 Put the spiced cream back on a medium heat. Once warm, add the cooked rice and peas and stir through to combine. Cook for 3 mins until everything is heated through.

3 Gently mix in the haddock, being careful to keep it in large flakes. Cook for a further 2 mins and check the seasoning – the smoked haddock will be quite salty, but a good grind of black pepper could be welcome.

4 Top the kedgeree with the boiled eggs and scatter over the coriander, then tip it into a large dish and take it to the table to serve.

Nutrition: *per serving*
kcal 885 fat 72g saturates 43g carbs 27g sugars 5g fibre 3g protein 30g salt 0.5g

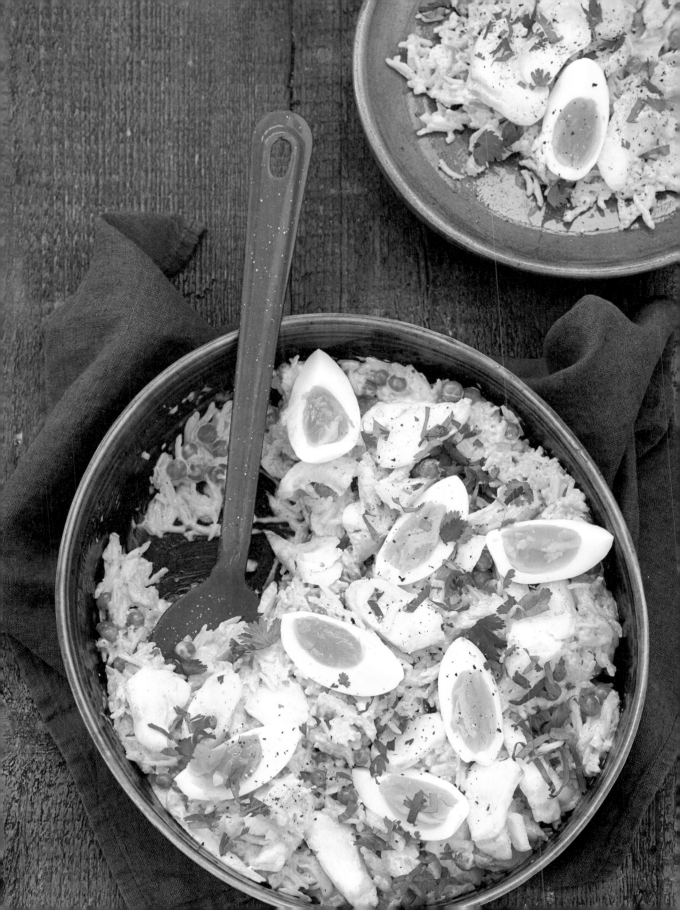

Healthy banana & peanut putter ice cream

Sweet cinnamon adds a subtle spice to this healthy ice cream.

🕐 PREP 10 mins plus freezing NO COOK 🍽 4

- 4 ripe bananas, chopped into 3cm chunks, then frozen
- 2 tbsp almond milk
- 1 tbsp organic peanut butter
- 1½ tsp ground cinnamon
- 1 tbsp dark chocolate, grated
- 1 tbsp flaked almonds

1 Tip the frozen bananas and almond milk into a blender. Blend together to create a smooth consistency. Add the peanut butter and cinnamon, and blend again. Taste and add more cinnamon, if you like.
2 Transfer to a freezer-proof container and freeze for 1 hr.
3 Take out of the freezer and serve with grated chocolate and flaked almonds sprinkled over.

Nutrition: *per serving*
kcal 169 fat 6g saturates 2g carbs 24g sugars 22g fibre 2g protein 3g salt 0g

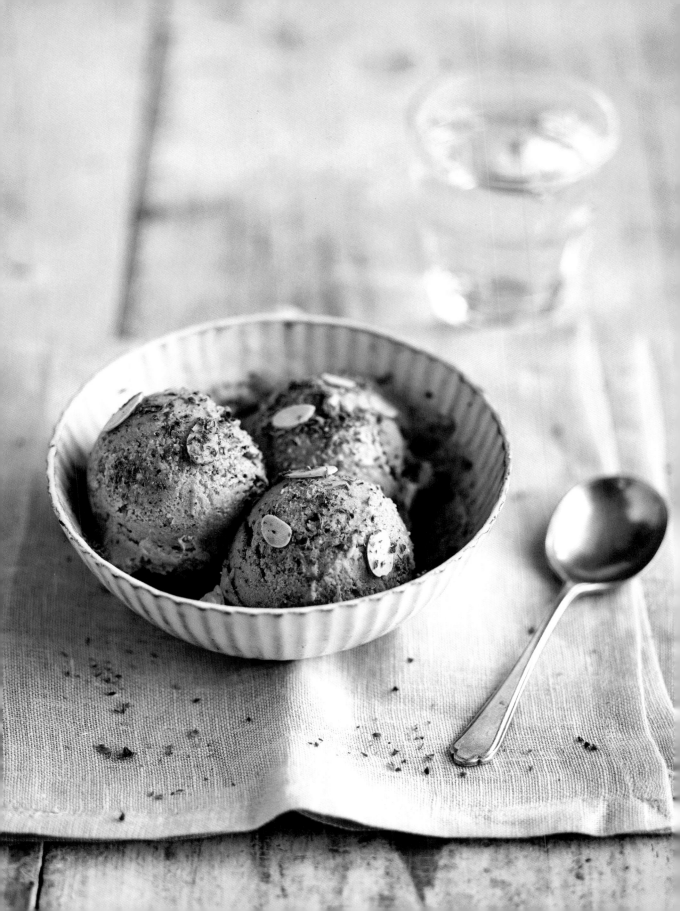

Index